P9-CND-814

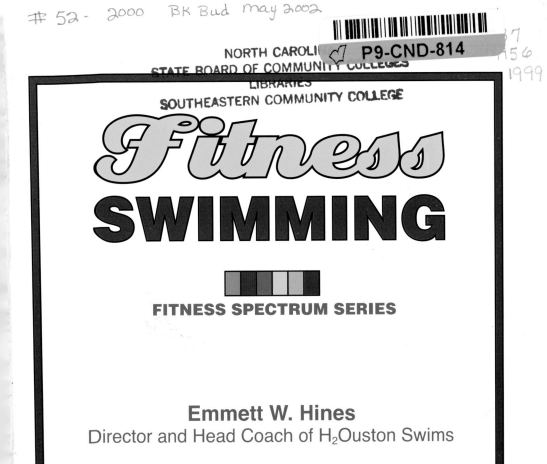

Fitness

SWIMMING

FITNESS SPECTRUM SERIES

Emmett W. Hines
Director and Head Coach of H₂Ouston Swims

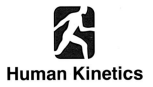

Human Kinetics

This book is dedicated to my family—
Peggy, Kalen, and Nolan Wolfgang—
who renew my joy and confidence day by day,
and my Mom and Dad for whom my respect and admiration continue to grow.

Library of Congress Cataloging-in-Publication Data

Hines, Emmett W., 1956-
    Fitness swimming / Emmett W. Hines.
        p. cm. -- (Fitness spectrum series)
        ISBN 0-88011-656-0 (pbk.)
        1. Swimming--Training.   2. Physical fitness.   I. Title.
    II. Series.
    GV837.7.H56   1999
    613.7'16--dc21   98-16314
                                                                   CIP

ISBN: 0-88011-656-0

Copyright © 1999 by Human Kinetics Publishers

Acquisitions Editor: Kenneth Mange; **Developmental Editor**: Andrew Smith; **Managing Editor**: Laura Hambly; **Assistant Editors**: John Wentworth, Phil Natividad; **Copyeditor**: Denelle Eknes; **Proofreader**: Debra Aglaia; **Graphic Designer**: Keith Blomberg; **Graphic Artist**: Sandra Meier; **Photo Editor**: Boyd LaFoon; **Cover Designer**: Jack Davis; **Photographer (cover)**: Dan Helms; **Photographer (interior)**: Sheila Baskett—unless otherwise noted; **Illustrator**: John Hatton

Human Kinetics books are available at special discounts for bulk purchase. Special editions or book excerpts can also be created to specification. For details, contact the Special Sales Manager at Human Kinetics.

Printed in Hong Kong   10   9   8   7   6   5   4   3   2   1

Human Kinetics
Web site: http://www.humankinetics.com/

United States: Human Kinetics, P.O. Box 5076, Champaign, IL 61825-5076
1-800-747-4457
e-mail: humank@hkusa.com

Canada: Human Kinetics, 475 Devonshire Road Unit 100, Windsor, ON N8Y 2L5
1-800-465-7301 (in Canada only)
e-mail: humank@hkcanada.com

Europe: Human Kinetics, P.O. Box IW14, Leeds LS16 6TR, United Kingdom
(44) 1132 781708
e-mail: humank@hkeurope.com

Australia: Human Kinetics, 57A Price Avenue, Lower Mitcham, South Australia 5062
(088) 277 1555
e-mail: humank@hkaustralia.com

New Zealand: Human Kinetics, P.O. Box 105-231, Auckland 1
(09) 523 3462
e-mail: humank@hknewz.com

Contents

Acknowledgments

Swimming is both an individual sport and a team sport. The success of the team relies chiefly on the performances of individual swimmers. Those swimmers, in turn, rely on the team swimmers, coaches, managers, and so on for training, facilities, instruction, motivation, inspiration, and everything else that allows them to prepare for and rise to the competitive occasion. As a coach of such a sport, I would be remiss if I did not thank and acknowledge those who have helped, supported, or inspired me along the way . . . so far . . .

Drew Berkman, for pointing me in the right direction at the right time. Coach Bill Boomer, who goes his own way and unselfishly allows others to follow and look over his shoulder from time to time. Coach Mike Collins, who serves constantly as an inspiration and role model. Rookie Dickenson, who gave me the freedom, time, and pool space to grow a Masters swimming program from scratch. Dr. Ken Forster for being a friend and co-conspirator. Coach Phil Hansel, who let me hang around enough to learn a lot. Coach Terry Laughlin, who helps it all make sense. Ed Lewis without whose support and confidence I would still have a real job. Coach Scott Rabalais for his kind words, friendship, and example. Leslie Ronacher for her moral support and bagels. Author Phil Whitten for his friendship and inspiration and for taking a chance on me. I must also acknowledge the swimmers of H_2Ouston Swims for motivating me, trusting me, and being receptive to new ideas.

I would also like to thank Coach Dick Bower, whose body of work provided me with the information about cruise intervals and cruise pace. In addition, the technique concepts expressed herein are the result of combining and distilling information from a wealth of sources; most notably, the work of Coaches Bill Boomer and Terry Laughlin forms the foundation, framework, and vital mass.

Finally, my parents, wife, and children are due loud and public acclaim for being patient and putting up with me while I try to save the world (or at least the swimming part of it).

PART I

PREPARING TO SWIM

Swimming is, arguably, the most popular of all fitness activities. Properly done, it can be most pleasurable, allowing the physical expression of fluidity and grace with power, speed, and stamina. Swimming offers a wealth of opportunity to condition the cardiovascular system while it tones and strengthens the body. As such, it can be an excellent tool for improving and maintaining lifelong fitness.

Improperly done, though, swimming can be an exhausting and excruciating struggle in which you perceive that you are hovering at the brink of drowning. Perhaps you are one of the estimated 98 percent of Americans who are unable to swim more than 500 yards without stopping. It is not physical conditioning that limits most people; it is their technique. They can swim, but their style causes them to waste so much energy that they fatigue and must stop long before they receive any aerobic benefit. For these people, swimming is more of a survival skill than a fitness tool.

You may be one of those swimmers who swims for extended periods, but are aware that you still have room for improvement. Perhaps you currently swim for fitness, triathlon, Masters competition, or for the pure pleasure of being in the water. Regardless, chances are that you are enviously aware that some swimmers around you are faster, more efficient, or look more experienced.

Swimming is inherently a technique-limited sport—more like golf in that respect than like running or cycling. As with golf, nearly anybody willing to spend the time and effort can learn and maintain the skills of excellent swimming—fluid, graceful swimming. The fitness payoff for such expenditures can be enormous. Few other activities offer a full-body workout with the prospect of participation well beyond the age where other sports are unthinkable.

However, few swimmers ever reach the fluid, graceful stage without following some road map, whether it be a coach, instructor, video, book, or combination thereof. Regardless of your ability level and your participation goals, it is my hope that this book will serve you as such a road map, starting or keeping you on course to a lifelong, pleasurable, and beneficial acquaintance with the water. I therefore lay the groundwork for your swim training in the first part of the book (chapters 1-5), including the following:

- Comparing the benefits of swimming to those of other fitness activities
- Helping you to choose the proper swimming equipment to fit your needs and offering suggestions on finding the best places to swim
- Testing your physical readiness to engage in a swim training program or to intensify an existing program
- Explaining the fundamentals of efficient swimming and presenting a progression of drills guaranteed to improve the efficiency of your freestyle stroke
- Adding information about warm-up, cool-down, and flexibility exercises

Swimming for Fitness

There is no other truly lifetime sport than swimming. Babies are born with a natural affinity for water and its womb-like feeling of security. Almost immediately there are opportunities for kids to maintain an acquaintance with the water. Mom and Tot or Waterbabies programs teach parents to make sure their kids' initial experiences with water are safe, comfortable, and encouraging. Real swimming lessons begin as early as age three, and in many areas of the country kids start swimming in races in summer leagues as early as age five. A person can stay involved in swimming programs such as United States Swimming (USS) age group and summer league swimming up to age 15, then move to high school swimming, college varsity and intramural swimming, Masters swimming, Senior Olympics, YMCA classes, and community lap swim classes. Many adults continue swimming literally until the day they die. It is common to see people in their 60s, 70s, or 80s swimming laps in lanes next to 20- or 30-year-old swimmers.

Swimming is enjoyed in its various forms by more Americans than any other sport. Certainly, some of the 60-million Americans who indicate that they participate in swimming are referring to one week last summer when they waded knee deep in the ocean and a wave got their suit wet. Yet, you have only to visit any pool with lane lines early in the morning, during lunch, or after work to know there is a huge number of fitness swimmers vying for lane space.

Chances are, if you ever go past knee deep, you fall into one of the following categories:

Novice swimmer.   You can swim one or two lengths of the pool without stopping, using the crawl stroke or breaststroke, and you wouldn't drown if you were to fall in the deep end. In fact, you could swim a couple hundred yards if your life depended on it, but probably have never swum more than 500 yards in one day.

Lap swimmer.   You swim a mile or more on a good day. You do your last few lengths pretty fast, just to top it off so you feel good and tired, or time a couple 50s if the pace clock is on. You swim freestyle well and maybe one more stroke well enough to do in public. We commonly refer to the largest segment of the fitness swimming public as lap swimmers. Every day millions of people head to a nearby pool for an hour or so of solitary laps.

Former competitive swimmer.   You have some competitive background—USS, Amateur Athletic Union (AAU), high school, or college. You swim (or swam) all four competitive strokes. Although you rarely swim more than 1,000 yards, you are usually good for a couple races at pool parties.

Competitor.   You're a participating triathlete or a Masters swimmer. You compete often or occasionally. You work out regularly and go 1,500 to 5,000 yards on a workout day. You do interval work and probably swim with other swimmers about your ability, or you belong to a Masters swim team.

Whichever group you are in, you will be able to use this book to increase your involvement in swimming, whether for fitness or competition. Novice swimmers will learn how the water affects their bodies and how to use physical principles to make getting to the other end less of a gauntlet. You will also learn to use swimming as a fitness tool. Lap swimmers will learn what it takes to look and move like an accomplished swimmer, with more efficient positions and motions. You will discover new ways to focus your training time so it is more productive. Former competitive swimmers will discover new information about swimming technique and conditioning that was not available during their earlier swimming years. Active competitors, like former competitors, will learn cutting-edge information about technique and training that they may only have caught snippets of from magazine articles or from coaches or training partners. This book will also give active competitors ideas for spending pool time efficiently when training on their own, whether at home or on the road.

Benefits of Swimming

Swimming is widely recognized by health and fitness professionals as a nearly perfect activity to improve aerobic fitness, flexibility, body strength, muscle tone, and coordination. Wear and tear on the body is an almost universal problem with any activity more strenuous than channel surfing. Swimming has the distinction of being the sport lowest in wear and tear.

Coaching and training practitioners in virtually every sport acknowledge the efficacy of water exercise in its various forms as an adjunct to their athletes' training. Whether it's a professional boxer using the natural resistance of water to make his punches more powerful, the Olympic 100-meter runner using water running to augment her sprint training, or the professional football or basketball player using water exercise in a physical therapy regimen, athletes in all sports are coming to water to improve their primary sports.

Swimming, quite simply, is the supreme form of water exercise. Challenging to the mind and the body, uplifting to the spirit and the flesh, swimming is a fascinating sport that can grab you, hold you, and keep you healthy for the rest of your life. "There are two things in existence that

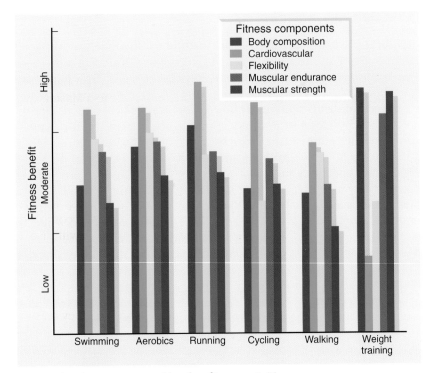

How swimming compares with other fitness activities.

nobody thinks are bad for you—swimming and yogurt," (Leonard Goodman in the *Wall Street Journal*).

Aerobic Conditioning

If you canvas the ranks of fitness swimmers, you will find that a common goal is to improve aerobic fitness. Exercise intended to improve aerobic fitness affects two related systems, the cardiovascular system and the muscular system, which have different conditioning components.

Cardiovascular Conditioning.
Any exercise that raises your heart rate higher than 120 beats per minute for longer than 20 minutes improves the condition of the cardiovascular system. The cardiovascular system is the well-known system of heart, lungs, and blood vessels that gets oxygen from the air you breathe into your lungs and transports it to the individual muscle cells where it will be used. Oxygen enters the lungs, with all the other crud you breathe in, and diffuses through the walls of huge numbers of capillaries and into your red blood cells. Through a maze of different-sized blood vessels, the heart pumps these red blood cells to the capillaries surrounding muscle cells and fibers, still carrying their precious cargo of oxygen. Here the transition from the cardiovascular system to the muscular system takes place.

Muscular System Aerobic Conditioning.
Once the cardiovascular system delivers the red blood cells to a muscle cell that requires more oxygen, the oxygen diffuses across the muscle cell membrane and into the cell, where it helps produce energy for muscle contractions. The term aerobic metabolism identifies a complex set of chemical interactions that take fats, carbohydrates, and oxygen and produce energy for exercise. Aerobic conditioning causes a variety of adaptations within the muscle cell that improves the cell's ability to perform work for extended periods.

Swimming properly involves a greater percentage of your body's muscle mass in aerobic exercise than any other popular activity. Cross-country skiing is the only other sport vying for this position.

Aerobic conditioning of any specific muscle occurs only when the exercise you are doing causes that muscle to contract repeatedly and consistently throughout your workout. No wonder the runner or cyclist who takes up swimming finds that, despite their excellent cardiovascular conditioning level, swimming a few laps leaves them fatigued. They have spent time aerobically conditioning the lower extremities but have done little or no conditioning of the torso and upper extremities.

Muscular Strength

Although swimming does not build huge, rippling muscles, even moderate-intensity distance swimming is excellent for improving strength and tone

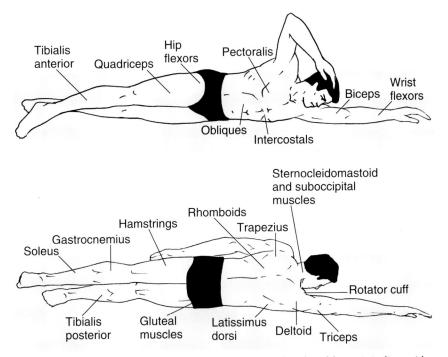

Muscles used in swimming: Neck muscles rotate the head and keep it in line with the spine. Muscles of the back, upper torso, and shoulders are used to transmit the large forces of trunk rotation to the stroking arm, and in recovering the arm after taking a stroke. Arm muscles help hold onto a spot in the water as the torso rotates past that spot. Lower torso muscles help accentuate and accelerate body roll. Muscles in the buttocks and legs are for kicking and initiating body roll.

in several muscles, especially torso, shoulder, and arm muscles. More experienced swimmers use high-intensity interval and sprint training to gain large increases in overall body strength. One of swimming's advantages is developing functional strength through the large ranges of motion swimmers used in the sport.

Flexibility

Inherent flexibility improvement may be one of the greatest benefits of swimming. It certainly is one of the largest factors allowing people to participate fully in the sport, well past ages where they must drop other sports. Because of the large ranges of motion swimmers use and the positions we ask the body to move through when executing proper strokes, we find that virtually all people who swim regularly become more flexible and supple. In addition, proper stroke technique builds on a series of plyometric contractions—motions that stretch a muscle just before applying the contractile force. This is similar to winding up before throwing a ball to stretch all the throwing muscles before they contract. Plyometric contractions increase flexibility and strength over time.

Body Composition

Much has been said over the years about whether swimming is a good way to get leaner. Like any form of exercise, the intensity with which you approach the sport has a lot to do with the results you get. One has only to look at the sleek, well-proportioned, long-muscled bodies of swimmers mounting the blocks at any swimming competition to know that swimming can produce a body you would be proud to wear almost nothing on. By the same token, there are plenty of people who go to the pool and just piddle around, applying the bare minimum of effort to slowly move from one end to the other. These people are likely to complain that swimming does nothing for them. After putting the same amount of effort into running, cycling, or any other sport, these people would, most likely, have the same complaint.

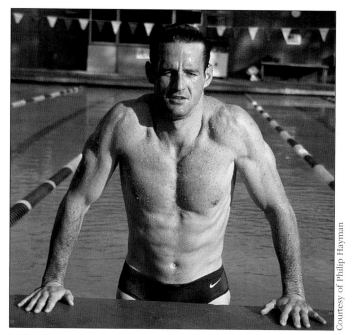

Courtesy of Philip Hayman

Swimming is a great way to attain a healthy body composition.

So, are you convinced? Swimming will be your next life challenge and passion. Now you need a swim suit and a few other goodies and you're off to find a swimmin' hole!

2

Getting Equipped

One appealing thing about swimming is the simplicity of equipping yourself. Very little is necessary to enjoy the sport. Yet, for those who like to own every conceivable bit of paraphernalia that you could apply to a sport, there is a variety available. Unfortunately, though, those who require great outlays of cash before feeling satisfied may be disappointed with this water sport.

Essential Equipment

For less than the cost of a cheap date you can have all you need to participate in the sport—swimsuit, goggles, cap, towel, and water bottle.

Swimsuit

Of all the things you might want for swimming pleasure, your suit is the most important. There are, in general, three worlds in the swimsuit universe—competitive suits (what you are looking for), fashion suits (what you see in *Sports Illustrated*), and monstrosities (what my grandmother wears at the beach).

The term competitive doesn't mean the suit is only for competition. It is a term used to describe the variety of suits that offer minimum drag in the water. If you are going to swim laps, this will be important. The key is to wear a suit that is comfortable, yet snugly fits your body, leaving no fabric loose to flap around in the water. When you are trying on a suit in the store, bear in mind that it will stretch one full size within your first few sessions in the pool. If in doubt, get one a bit small rather than too big.

Virtually all workout suits are made of Lycra. If you stick with major brands, you'll get a 128-grade Lycra fabric that is more chlorine and mold resistant than cheaper suits—well worth the extra expense. If you swim daily, get at least two suits. Putting on a cold, wet suit, especially first thing in the morning, is about as fun as watching a cat cough up a fur ball.

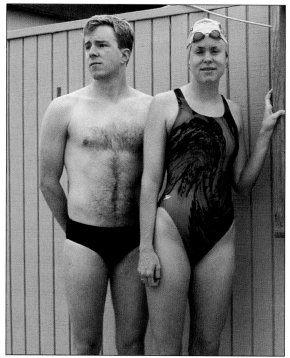

Competitive swim suits.

Women's suits usually run $50 to $60 for top-quality suits in the latest prints, and men's suits will be about $22 to $27. In most swim shops you'll find a rack of discontinued prints of the same high-quality suits for about half the price of the latest prints.

Women's Suits.   Men and women were not created equal. Men can usually wear any men's suit bearing their size on the label. For women the size printed on the tag is merely a starting point. The backs and straps on women's suits come in a variety of configurations. Because swimming involves so much range of motion of the arms and shoulders, the way any particular back style fits you and the way you move will be important. When trying on suits in the store, be sure to stretch into full streamline position and move your arms around to see if the suit will hamper your motion. You may go through several styles from different manufacturers before you find the style that works best for you.

For women it is particularly important not to get too big a suit. A suit that is not snug enough will catch large amounts of water and act as a drag chute. In general, if the shoulder straps will stretch higher than your ears, the suit is too big. Women have the option of a one-piece workout suit or a two-piece workout bikini.

Men's Suits.   In the case of men, a suit is a suit is a suit. Once you decide which size fits you best, you will be happy with any suit from the major manufacturers. However, some guys just can't bring themselves to wear one of those skimpy little racing suits. Several manufacturers offer a line of fuller cut suits with five-inch side panels instead of the standard three-inch side panels. If this won't suffice either and you've got to have a pair of beach baggies, do yourself a favor and sew the pockets shut so they don't balloon up like little drag chutes as you plod down the lane.

Choosing, Using, and Tweaking Goggles

Goggles maintain a small pocket of air directly in front of the eye and hold a transparent lens that allows near-normal vision. They also protect the swimmer's eyeballs from the discomfort of prolonged exposure to chlorine.

Modern materials have made inexpensive, compact, lightweight, comfortable goggles a reality, and a growing swimming population, willing to part with its cash, has spawned a cornucopia of goggle styles to choose from. However, only a few of those styles are likely right for you. Aside from your swimsuit, there is nothing within your control that will more greatly affect your comfort and appreciation for swimming than the right pair of goggles. Here are a few things to consider when choosing your perfect pair of goggles.

- **Shape.** There are two basic shapes for goggles, which I refer to as sort-of-round and more-oval. If you find one pair of oval goggles that works well for you, most likely, any goggle that works well for you will be more-oval. The same kind of thinking also applies if you find that a pair of sort-of-round goggles works well.

- **Gaskets.** The gasket is the soft material around the eyecup of the goggle that fills the voids in the goggle to face union. There are several types to choose from: foam, silicone, polyvinyl, or none. For simplicity, ease of care, and length of service, none tops the list. Popular Swedish-style goggles have no gasket, allowing the most streamlined, face-hugging fit. However, if your face wasn't molded to the same contour as the goggle, you will be happier with a gasketed goggle. Solid silicone or polyvinyl gaskets make a good seal if the goggle is the correct shape for your face and offer excellent resistance to microbial growth. Foam gaskets, although more forgiving in making a leak-proof seal, are prone to grow low-order life forms if not properly maintained.

- **Antifog.** This is a highly touted selling point for a variety of goggle styles. Goggles fog up when moisture in the air trapped in the eyecup condenses on the inside surface of the goggle from the relatively cool water around the goggle. Many goggles on the market tout antifog properties. I have yet to encounter, through experience or anecdote, any better antifog system than good ole American spit. A thin coating of saliva on the inside of the eyecup keeps it from fogging for a long time.

- **Goggles and contact lenses.** Many contact lens wearers are afraid to wear their lenses with goggles. However, you are less likely to lose a lens while swimming than you are while taking them out and putting them back in. Once you become accustomed to wearing goggles, you will be much happier if you keep your lenses in when swimming.

- **Prescription goggles.** For those who have a hard time making their way around on land without glasses, there is still hope of seeing the pace clock. Check with your optometrist about prescription goggles or prescription inserts for your goggles. There are some corrective-lens goggles available through swim shops or catalogs. Although you may not find your exact prescription, you most likely can find a pair that allows you to read a pace clock from across the pool.

Finally, once you do find your personal perfect goggle, buy several pairs. Murphy has a law. I don't recall the exact wording, but it has something to do with the availability, at any point in the future, of the only goggle style that fits *your* face.

Le Chapeau du Natation (Cap)

For any person whose hair is more than a few inches long, a proper swimming cap is necessary. Caps can serve many purposes, including

- keeping hair out of your eyes, nose, and mouth;
- affording less water resistance than hair;

- keeping your hair from absorbing too much chlorine;
- coordinating with your swimming ensemble; and
- proclaiming your affiliation.

There are three common materials for caps: latex, silicone, and Lycra. Latex caps are the most popular, least expensive, and fit the most swimmers. Silicone caps are more expensive, last longer (unless you get even a slight tear, in which case they are instant history), are harder to keep properly in place, and work well for fewer swimmers. Lycra caps are the least popular, most expensive, look funky, and don't protect your hair at all. I'm not sure why there is a market for them.

Regardless of what kind of cap you use, dry it thoroughly after each use. Dust it lightly with baby powder before you store it. Avoid leaving it wadded up in the bottom of your bag or in a hot car.

Water Bottle

Despite being immersed in cool water, your body still perspires when you swim and you are constantly blowing off water vapor as you breathe. Replenishing this water is vital to a safe and productive workout. Drink

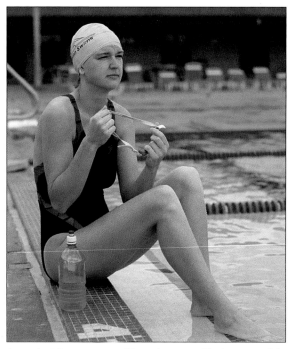

A modest investment will equip you with the essentials for swimming.

before you get thirsty and drink more than you think you need. Even if it is an old gallon milk jug full of tap water, bring this precious elixir of life to the poolside.

Other Equipment

For the person who doesn't feel complete until surrounded by equipment and gadgets, there is plenty of additional stuff available to complement the basics. Here is some equipment that is not essential but can come in handy with some workouts.

- **Training fins.** If you are following the workouts in this book, you will want at least one pair of training fins. Fins extend your foot and leg, making your kick more efficient and speedier. They also help increase ankle flexibility, increase leg strength, and activate more muscle mass. Most are made of natural rubber, although some are made of high-density, heat-treated polyurethane and will last forever. You might want a pair of short training fins (blade length of one or two inches) and another pair of normal-size training fins (blade is roughly the same length as your foot). Avoid rigid fins, blades wider than one and one-half times the width of your foot, and blades longer than your foot.

- **Hand paddles.** Properly used, hand paddles help you learn what it feels like to hold onto a spot in the water. In much the same way flippers enlarge your effective kicking surface, paddles enlarge your effective pulling surface. Paddles with large holes for water to pass through allow you to still feel water pressure on your palms. Paddles that are more than slightly larger than your hands can be rough on your shoulders.

- **Kickboard.** Kickboards are rigid foam boards designed to hold your upper body and head at or higher than the surface while kicking with your legs, forcing you to kick uphill to some extent. The kicking drills in this book are without a kickboard, as this promotes a more balanced position.

- **Pace clock, training watch, goggle clock.** Most workouts are organized in an interval training format that requires a visible timing device. If the pool you frequent does not have a pace clock, you will want to provide a timing device. The ideal is a portable 15-inch analog pace clock with sweep second hand and minute hand. The face is numbered from 5 to 60 in 5-second jumps with small tick marks for each second in between.

  An alternative to a pace clock is a sports timer watch. Look for one with multiple stopwatch functions, including lap split memory with countdown and countup interval timer. Two drawbacks to using a watch-type timer are that you can't see it while you are swimming, and recording lap splits requires you to reach over with your other hand and press a button, thereby slowing you down. However, you can't beat the portability of a watch.

There is a miniature stopwatch called a Time-Window (about $30) that attaches to the front of your goggle so your elapsed time is always in your field of view without interfering with your distance vision. Simply pressing its case starts, stops, or resets the device.

- **Heart rate monitor.** A monitor with a watch-style display and sensor that straps around your chest is the most accurate, but many people find them uncomfortable for extended use. Before investing in any heart rate monitor, borrow one to see if it suits you.

- **Electronic stroke monitor.** A stroke monitor is a sports watch that senses and counts each stroke as you take it; keeps track of time; calculates swimming speed, distance per stroke, cycling rate; and has a stroke efficiency index. If you want swimming efficiency but you hate counting strokes, you're going to end up owning one.

- **Antichlorine chemicals.** Modern science has spawned a variety of antichlorine shampoos, soaps, and body washes that work surprisingly well to remove chlorine from your hair and skin.

- **Cold equipment.** During all but the fairest weather, most avid swimmers bring warm clothing to the pool. Pullovers and parkas or big, thick thirsty towels fill the bill here.

- **Equipment bag.** So, you took this book to the local swim shop and said, "I'll have one of each, two of some." You now have a pile of stuff to schlep back and forth. Invest your last couple of sawbucks in two good swim bags. First, get a nylon mesh drawstring bag for the wet pool toys (kickboard, flippers, and paddles). Then, get a conventional workout bag for the usual locker-room stuff. It should have one or two external mesh pockets for damp suits and goggles and a waterproof compartment for wet towels. A waterproof bottom also comes in handy around constantly wet pool decks.

Where to Swim

As with any activity, the environment affects your enjoyment, influencing how often you participate and how long you stick with it. Sometimes, you have little choice in where you swim. If there's only one swimming hole available and only one hour of the day for lap swimming, then you have to make due. Usually though, you will have a variety of swimming options from which to choose.

ADDING UP THE COSTS

So, let me sum up the costs for what you will need to start swimming. As with most things, you can spend a small amount, just getting the basics, or you can go nuts and get everything possible. Let's start by looking at the basic costs.

LOW BUDGET COSTS

Item	Cost
Suit	$15 (men) $30 (women)
Goggles	$4
Cap	$1
Water bottle	$0 (old milk jug)
Towel	$0 (Thanks Motel 6)

For you equipment fanatics out there, here are the costs you are looking at.

HIGH BUDGET COSTS

Item	Cost
Suit	$15 to $27 (men) $30 to $60 (women)
Goggles	$4 to $35
Cap	$1 to $13
Water bottle	$0 to $8
Towel	$0 to $30
Kickboard	$10 to $28
Hand paddles	$10 to $20
Polyurethane fins	$75 to $85
Short fins	$30 to $40
Electronic stroke monitor	$80
Heart rate monitor	$90 to $210
Wrist sport timer	$25 to $200
Analog pace clock	$140 to $255
Sweatshirt	$12 to $30
Swimmer's parka	$80 to $100
Antichlorine soap, shampoo	$10 to $15
Mesh swim bag	$10 to $15
Duffel swim bag	$15 to $50

Pool Swimming

Once you are fully equipped, where do you go to put all your new stuff to best use? Not all pools are conducive to swimming laps. In general, there are three common lap pool configurations, long course, short course, and odd-length pools.

The most common lap pool configuration in the United States is referred to as short course. A short-course pool is either 25 yards or 25 meters long and will have from 4 to 10 lanes that are 5 to 9 feet wide.

In many facilities, size constraints dictate a smaller pool. Common in many hotel, motel, and fitness facilities are 20-yard pools, and from time to time you'll even encounter a 15-yard pool. If you have a good push-off with a streamlined glide and an efficient stroke, you won't get to swim many strokes before it is time to turn again.

The lanes in a long-course pool are 50 meters. This is the length of a true Olympic-size pool (95% of pools touted to be Olympic pools are, in fact, much smaller—it seems that hotel and motel owners and apartment complex operators think anything with a line on the bottom is fit for Olympic pursuits). Most long-course pools are either 25 yards or 25 meters wide so that, during some periods or seasons, the lane lines can be installed across the pool to allow short-course swimming.

The only requirements for a lap pool are clean, clear water at least three feet deep and lap lanes delineated by floating, wave-quelling lane markers. Wave-quelling lane markers are tightly stretched cables with three- to five-inch diameter floats and discs that run the length of the pool. In addition to defining the space for swimming laps, lane markers absorb most surface waves that hit them. Without these, swimming laps while other people use the pool can be dangerous from the standpoint of head-to-head collisions and unpleasant from the standpoint of choppy, turbulent water.

Swimming Without Walls

As a variation on lap swimming, some parts of the country have many swimmers who eschew the black line and lane markers for a more natural setting. If your swimming routine is confined to pools, you are missing a world of aquatic adventure. Virtually anywhere you can find clean water over 55 degrees, there are sure to be some open-water swimming enthusiasts. Although many people prefer to strike out on their own, experts agree that you should always swim in a properly supervised and patrolled open-water swimming area or with a buddy of roughly your speed. Although open-water swimming is a safe way to log many unfettered miles, it is also a good way to get into trouble on your own, especially if you are swimming in an unfamiliar area or in conditions you aren't used to. Properly supervised, open-water swimming gives the sport a whole new face. Try an ocean, lake, or quarry swim sometime. This is where true distance swimming takes place—everything else is just practice.

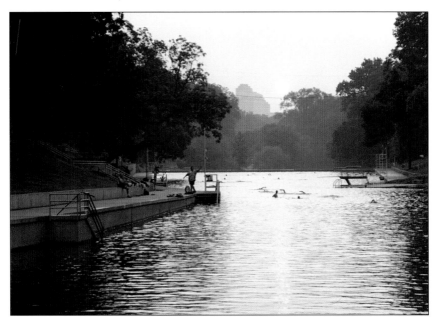

Everyone needs a change of pace and scenery at some point. Getting out of the pool and into the outdoors is a fun way to get a good workout, but be sure to swim with a buddy or a group.

Other Swimming Environment Considerations

There are a couple other issues about which a little knowledge will make your swimming experience more enjoyable.

Water Temperature.   Depending on the types of activities a pool is used for, management usually has a goal temperature from 76 to 88 degrees. The 78 to 82 degrees Fahrenheit considered optimal for lap swimming may seem warm if you aren't usually aware of water tempera-ture. However, water removes heat from your body more rapidly than air does. When they first hop in, 78 degrees will seem cool to most people, but as soon as you have been moving for a while it'll feel just fine. Water over 82 degrees can be uncomfortably warm while working out, and in water higher than 85 degrees you risk getting badly overheated when doing a strenuous workout. On the other end of the spectrum, most people can adapt well to temperatures as low as the mid 60s as long as they keep moving fast enough to maintain body temperature.

Depending on the physical plant capabilities, pool temperatures may be stable or variable. Indoor pools are usually well controlled within a degree or two. Outdoor pool temperatures are affected more by the weather, but in some parts of the country outdoor pools operate year-round, heated with gas, solar, or geothermal systems in the winter and cooled by aeration or geothermal systems in the summer. Open water, of course, is purely subject to Mother Nature's whims.

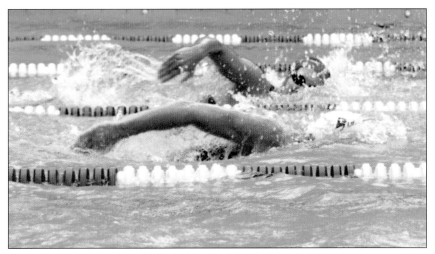

Water temperature of 78 to 82 degrees makes any swim much more comfortable.

Chlorine. One common complaint the unenlightened have is chlorine. The chlorine most pool operators use to maintain sanitized water will attach itself to your skin and hair, and once attached, it is tenacious. The people you contact during the rest of the day will know you're a swimmer by the Eau de Cement Pond fragrance you sport. Consistent exposure to chlorine can also make hair feel and act like straw.

Common sense and the right toiletries can nip these problems in the bud. When you first wet yourself, your skin and hair absorb water. If you take a shower before getting in the pool, there is little chlorine in the tap water to absorb. If you hop straight into the pool without the shower, your hair and skin absorb lots of pool water, in which the chlorine level is typically 2 to 10 times as high as tap water. Take your pick. That was the common sense part. In addition to showering before hitting the pool, you can rub a dab of conditioner into your hair before putting on your cap. In any case, if you are fussy about your hair, wear a cap.

If you follow these few suggestions and use the chlorine-removal products mentioned earlier, you should be able to hide the fact that you are a swimmer from the rest of the world. Then again, why would you want to?

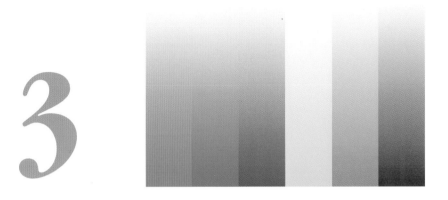

3

Checking Your Swimming Fitness

You have rendered unto Caesar in return for a bag full of swim goodies and you have located a near-perfect swimming hole. There remains one task to complete before you launch yourself headlong into the blue and start stroking with reckless abandon. You must get a feel for the level of swimming fitness at which you will begin your new training program.

My operating definition of fitness for swimming is as follows: Fitness is the ability to express the technique you have developed, over whatever time you choose, at whatever intensity you choose. Fitness is specific to the task at hand. A person may have a high level of fitness for distance running yet be completely unfit for swimming. A person might be fit for swimming long distances yet unfit for sprinting one length of the pool.

The terms health and fitness are often used in the same breath, as if they were inseparable. Although it is true that if you have high-fitness levels for a wide range of physical pursuits you have a greater likelihood of being healthy, the converse is not necessarily true. You can be healthy in the sense of being illness and injury free, yet be completely unprepared for any prolonged or intense physical exertion.

Measuring Your Health and Fitness

The next couple of pages are a self-test questionnaire to identify any contraindications for increased physical activity. This is then followed by a specific swimming test to do in the pool. These two tests will help to determine whether to consult a physician before beginning your swimming program and at what level you should start.

Choose the number that best describes you in each of these 10 areas; then add up your score. The results tell whether your base condition is high, average, or low.

ASSESSING YOUR SWIMMING READINESS

Cardiovascular Health: **Which statement best describes your cardiovascular condition? This is a critical safety check before you enter any vigorous activity. (Warning: If you have a cardiovascular disease history, start the swimming programs in this book only after receiving clearance from your doctor—then only with close supervision by a fitness instructor.)**

No history of heart or circulatory problems	____ (3)
Past ailments treated successfully	____ (2)
Such problems exist but no treatment required	____ (1)
Under medical care for cardiovascular illness	____ (0)

Injuries: **Which statement best describes your current injuries? This is a test of your musculoskeletal readiness to start a swimming program. (Warning: If your injury is temporary, wait until it is cured before starting the program. If it is chronic, adjust the program to fit your limitations.)**

No current injury problems	____ (3)
Some pain in activity but not limited by it	____ (2)
Level of activity limited by the injury	____ (1)
Unable to do much strenuous training	____ (0)

Illnesses: **Which statement best describes your current illnesses? Certain temporary or chronic conditions will delay or disrupt your swimming program. (See warning under Injuries.)**

No current illness problems	____ (3)
Some problem in activity but not limited by it	____ (2)
Level of activity limited by the illness	____ (1)
Unable to do much strenuous training	____ (0)

Age: **In which age group do you fall? In general, the younger you are, the less time you have spent slipping out of shape.**

Age 20 or younger   ____ (3)
Age 21 to 29   ____ (2)
Age 30 to 39   ____ (1)
Age 40 and older   ____ (0)

Weight: **Which range best describes how close you are to your definition of ideal weight? Excess fat, which can be layered on thin people too, is a sign of unhealthy inactivity. Of course, being underweight isn't ideal either.**

Within 2 pounds of your ideal weight   ____ (3)
Less than 10 pounds higher or lower than your ideal   ____ (2)
11 to 19 pounds higher or lower than your ideal   ____ (1)
20 or more pounds higher or lower than your ideal   ____ (0)

Resting Pulse Rate: **Which range describes your current resting pulse rate, which is your pulse upon waking in the morning before getting out of bed? The heart of a fit person normally beats more slowly and efficiently than an unfit heart.**

Less than 60 beats per minute   ____ (3)
61 to 69 beats per minute   ____ (2)
70 to 79 beats per minute   ____ (1)
80 or more beats per minute   ____ (0)

Smoking: **Which statement describes your smoking history and current habits? Smoking is the major demon behind ill health that you can control.**

Never a smoker   ____ (3)
Once a smoker, but quit   ____ (2)
An occasional, social smoker now   ____ (1)
A regular, heavy smoker now   ____ (0)

Most Recent Swim: **Which statement best describes your swimming within the last month? The best single measure of how well you will swim in the near future is what you have swum in the recent past.**

Swam nonstop for more than 20 minutes   ____ (3)
Swam nonstop for 10 to 20 minutes   ____ (2)
Swam nonstop for 5 to 10 minutes   ____ (1)
Swam for less than 5 minutes or not at all   ____ (0)

Swimming Background: **Which statement best describes your swimming history? Swimming fitness isn't long lasting, but swimming technique, the dominant factor in swimming ability, is long lasting. The fact that you have been involved in swimming in the past is a good sign that you can do it again.**

Trained for swimming within the last year	____ (3)
Trained for swimming 1 to 2 years ago	____ (2)
Trained for swimming more than 2 years ago	____ (1)
Never trained formally for swimming	____ (0)

Related Activities: **Which statement best describes your participation in other aerobic activities? Continuous activities such as running, cross-country skiing, and bicycling help build a good foundation for swimming. Nonaerobic activities, such as weightlifting and stop-and-go sports like tennis, don't contribute as well.**

Regularly practice continuous aerobic activity	____ (3)
Sometimes practice continuous aerobic activity	____ (2)
Practice nonaerobic or stop-and-go sports	____ (1)
Not regularly active	____ (0)

Total score

After determining your total score, use the following scales to interpret the score.

20 or more = You rate high in health and fitness for a beginning swimmer. You can probably handle training sessions in the pool lasting 45 minutes or longer at a moderate pace with short rest periods.

10 to 19 = Your score is average. You may need to take longer rest breaks during a training session.

Less than 10 = Your score is below average. You may need to take frequent, longer breaks and swim more slowly. Beginning a new physical activity when you are at a low fitness level can be frustrating if your expectations are too high. If you have been inactive for some time, you should count your initial trips to the pool as major accomplishments even if you get tired easily or feel pooped. Moving from inactivity into a fitness activity is a big change that takes a while for your body to get used to. Keep after it though, because the lower your initial fitness level the greater your rewards will be in the near future.

Testing Your Swimming Fitness

OK, it's time to dispense with the theoretical pencil and paper stuff and get your new bathing suit, cap, and goggles wet. Your entrance exam is about to begin, but you can't do it while you are sitting there in that chair, so off you go to the pool.

This test is called a T-15 test. It is a 15-minute timed swim for distance. The idea is to see how far you can swim in 15 minutes. This test is an excellent practical indicator of your swimming ability. The ability to swim efficiently is considered 70 percent technique and only 30 percent conditioning. This test is an ideal way to assess your combined technique and conditioning levels at the same time.

A person may have a high overall fitness level for a variety of sports, yet, lacking proper swimming technique, might not be able to swim far in 15 minutes because the energy expenditure on every lap is high. On the other hand, consider a person who was at one time an elite-level competitive swimmer but has been sedentary for 10 years and is now in poor condition. They may swim farther on this test because their technique is excellent, allowing them to spend little energy on each lap.

For a swimming training program to be enjoyable and productive, the training regimen you undertake must enhance both elements of swimming ability—technique and conditioning. That's why you bought this book, isn't it? Congratulations, you are off to a great start.

T-15 SWIM

1. Swim any stroke or combination of strokes as far as possible in 15 minutes. You must count your laps. (A lap in a pool is two lengths and means, like on a running track, getting back to where you started. In a 25-yard pool, one lap is 50 yards; in a 50-meter pool, one lap is 100 meters.) Strive for an even pace throughout the swim. Avoid speeding up at the end of the swim. During the swim, if you need to stop and rest for short periods, you may do so. However, the clock keeps ticking and these rest periods are part of your elapsed time.

2. At the end of the swim, finish the lap you are on when 15:00 ticks by. Note your elapsed time when you complete that lap. This means you will have an elapsed time a bit *over* 15:00. (For example, near the end of the swim, you arrive at the wall and the pace clock shows you have been swimming for 14:40. You need to swim one more lap. When you complete that lap the clock shows 15:30. Now you are done.)

3. Upon completing the swim, take your immediate heart rate (IHR) reading. If you have a heart rate monitor, use your first stable reading. Otherwise, take a manual heart rate (more about heart rates and how to take them in part II).

Once you complete your swim, record and save four pieces of information, as shown in the following table. (The figures in this table provide a sample of possible outcomes for the T-15 test. They are not a guideline for you to shoot for.)

Sample Record for T-15 Swim

Information to record	Sample distance and time
Number of yards (or meters) you swam	950
Your IHR after the swim	150
Elapsed time of the swim	15:30
T-15 cruise pace per 100 yards (look up in table on page 176)	1:37.8

Once you have recorded the information, swim or tread water easily for at least five minutes to cool down. (Hint: To easily record information poolside, cut up a Tyvek envelope—you know, the ones you can't tear—into several three-by-five-inch pieces. Tyvek is waterproof, and you can write on it easily with a number-2 pencil.)

The last item you record is your cruise pace—your average pace per 100 yards during the swim. This is the fastest pace you can swim for an extended time, and it indicates your combined swimming fitness and ability level. The following table provides guidelines on what fitness and ability levels correspond to a range of cruise paces.

Estimates for Fitness and Ability Level at Various Cruise Pace Speeds

Cruise pace per 100 yards	Combined fitness and ability level
1:20 or less	Superior
1:21-1:40	High
1:41-2:00	Average
2:01-2:30	Below average
2:31+	Low

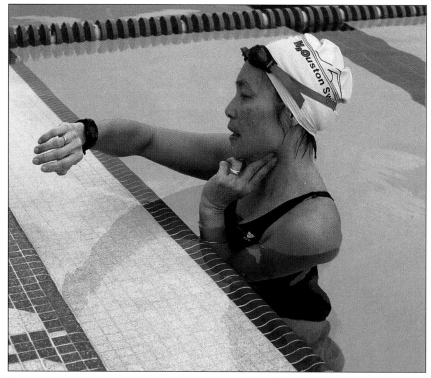

Be sure to take your heart rate immediately after finishing the T-15 swim test.

Retesting

The T-15 swim is a test you can repeat often, perhaps once per week. There are three ways to note an improvement in your T-15 performance: If you swim at a faster average pace (T-15 Cruise Pace Per 100 Chart in appendix A), if you swim the same pace but show a lower IHR, or if you have a lower average stroke count (as you read this book and start doing some practices you will become aware of how many strokes you take to swim a length of the pool). Over the long haul, the best way to have the largest improvements in your T-15 swims is to focus your efforts on technique and efficiency.

After you have swum a few T-15s, you will feel confident enough to do T-20 swims. The concept and execution are the same as the T-15, except that you use a 20-minute swim time instead of 15 minutes. Eventually you'll move up to T-30 swims. Use the T-20 and T-30 charts in appendix A to judge your progress in the T-20 and T-30 tests. Look in chapter 14 for a blank chart you can photocopy to keep track of your T-15, T-20, and T-30 swim performances, so you can easily see your progress over time.

Swimming Golf

Swimming golf is more a test of technical ability than conditioning, and you can use it as a benchmark to indicate technique improvement over time. The rules are as follows:

1. Swim 50 yards (or meters), counting the total number of strokes you take in the 50 (count once for each hand as it enters the water in front of you). For example, if you are in a 25-yard pool and you take 21 strokes on the first length followed by 22 strokes coming back, your total is 43.

2. At the end of the swim, note your elapsed swim time in seconds. Let's say the swim took 47 seconds.

3. Add the number of strokes to the number of seconds. The total is your score for that swim. Add the 43 strokes to the 47 seconds for a total of 90.

4. Take as much rest as you want, and repeat from number 1, this time attempting to get a lower score (hence the name swimming golf).

5. Do this four times and average your scores. This is your par for next time. Your scores are 90, 89, 89, 88. Your average, or new par, is 89.

Better swimmers get lower stroke counts and fewer seconds than less accomplished swimmers. In a typical Masters group, 50-yard freestyle golf scores can easily range from the high 40s to over 100. Try to lower scores by decreasing your stroke count and your swim times. Start by lowering stroke count. Once you get comfortable with a lower stroke count, then increase the turnover rate without adding any strokes. Every time you hit a new, lower score you have become a better swimmer.

If you swim with others, swimming golf allows people of different abilities to compete head to head. Two experienced swimming golfers can take turns swimming 50s and compare their score for each swim to their personal par, keeping score over several 50s, just like cart-driving, beer-drinking golf. Jotting down numbers on those little Tyvek sheets between swims makes keeping track of scores easy. Look in chapter 14 for a blank chart you can photocopy to keep track of your swimming golf performances, so you can easily see your progress over time.

4

Swimming the Right Way

Let's face it, the human body wasn't designed for swimming. However, the advance of civilization has allowed those of us at the top of the food chain to spend idle time toying with nature. As such, we have made modest progress in aquatic ambulation.

Swimming Is a Technique Sport

Compared with swimming, running is an activity that the human body was designed to do. Running and, to a large extent, cycling involve simple and instinctive patterns and ranges of motion. Athletes have found that in both sports speed, endurance, and technique all improve dramatically by simply training more or harder. This is why most running and cycling training regimens concentrate chiefly on conditioning activities rather than technique activities.

Swimming is an entirely different animal. People think of swimming in much the same way as running and cycling—get in and do whatever you do longer, harder, and faster and you'll become a better swimmer. To some degree this is true. However, swimming is the most complex set of repetitive, rhythmic motions that exists in sport. More muscle groups must move through more ranges of motion in flawless coordination than in any other repetition-intensive activity. The coordination required to execute fluid, efficient swimming strokes is almost beyond comprehension. Also, because swimming motions and positions are not natural, we find that just doing it isn't enough to improve technique.

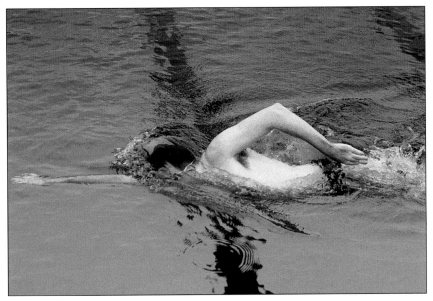

Just doing more and harder training won't make you a faster swimmer—just a better *conditioned* swimmer. Learning proper technique is more important than conditioning for long-term improvement.

What this book offers is a tried and true method to sharpen freestyle swimming skills you already have and add new aquatic skills to your arsenal. This is done within the framework of practice and conditioning exercises presented in a graduated workout format.

Freestyle Swimming

By far, the most popular swimming style for fitness is the stroke known as *freestyle*. In competitive swimming there are four regulation strokes— butterfly, backstroke, breaststroke, and freestyle. The first three have specific and constraining rules that govern how you swim the strokes. By contrast, according to the rules, you may swim a freestyle event in any manner you choose, as long as you complete the distance without touching the bottom, sides, or lane ropes.

Most swimmers choose some variation of the crawl stroke for swimming freestyle events. This is because, when swum properly, it is the fastest, most efficient method of moving through the water. Thus, the term freestyle has become the standard term for the crawl. In swimming circles, the term "crawl" is virtually nonexistent.

In addition to being the fastest stroke, it is the easiest to teach and learn. This probably explains why freestyle is the overwhelming favorite of fitness swimmers. I concentrate on refining and training the freestyle stroke in this book. However, many concepts, fundamentals, and drills I detail in this chapter and build into the workouts in the following chapters also apply to one or more of the other three strokes.

Water Resistance

Water is roughly 1,000 times denser than air. Unlike running, in which most of the energy you apply to the road ends up as forward motion, you use the majority of the energy you expend in swimming to overcome resistance. World-class swimmers are, at best, 9 percent efficient. At most, 9 percent of the energy they expend applies to forward progress. They spend the other 91 percent overcoming resistance in various forms. Less accomplished swimmers are not as efficient; perhaps as little as 2 percent of their effort becomes forward progress. It makes sense then to employ much of our practice time learning how to combat (or, more accurately, *avoid*) these unrelenting forces of nature.

Three Types of Resistance

There are three major types of resistance acting externally on the swimmer's body as it moves through water.

1. **Form drag** is the resistance that results from the shape of an object moving through the water. Reducing the frontal surface area that meets the oncoming flow of water reduces form drag. This means always keeping the body balanced as close to horizontal as possible, and keeping it long and narrow while swimming. It also means eliminating unnecessary motions. If you are perfectly streamlined, any motion you make increases form drag, so avoid movement beyond the minimum necessary to propel yourself. Just as a builder shapes long, tapered hulls instead of flat, square hulls on a racing boat, we want to taper the form and profile of the human body as it travels through the water and keep it that way. A swimmer that understands and applies the concepts of balance and streamlining can dramatically reduce form drag.

2. **Wave drag** is the resistance a body encounters as a result of creating a wake—just like a boat does. For the body to move forward through the surface, it must move water out of the way in the form of a wave

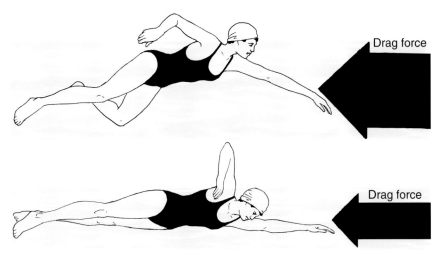

The largest source of resistance in swimming is form drag. Reducing the frontal surface area that meets the oncoming flow of water can dramatically reduce form drag.

traveling away from the moving body. Creating this wave takes energy—all of it supplied by the swimmer. The amount of energy required depends largely on how far the water must travel to get out of the way of the moving body. The wider a path the swimmer cuts through the surface, the bigger the wave and the more energy the swimmer spends overcoming wave drag. In freestyle and backstroke we look for positions that cut a narrower path through the surface by maximizing the time we spend on the side rather than flat on the back or stomach.

3. **Surface drag** is resistance caused by the frictional force of a moving body in water. We can reduce surface drag not through technique but through preparation and equipment. Properly fitting swimsuits and swimming caps help achieve this result. Shaving body hair or wearing a special competition suit that uses new high-tech materials to reduce water absorption will also reduce surface drag.

Minimizing Drag

Perhaps the single biggest tip to minimizing resistance from all sources is, first, to be aware of it, then act on that awareness. Use your senses to give yourself feedback about where you are fighting the water. Listen for splashing or kerplunking sounds and try to eliminate them. Feel for smooth, flowing movements of all parts of your body instead of bulldozing movements. You are trying to slip through the water rather than plow through it. Look for large or numerous bubbles in the water around you—

a sure sign of turbulence-causing actions. We gear much of our training to help you make adjustments to reduce or eliminate these resistance indicators and the motions and positions that cause them.

The fitness swimming skill drills and training approach in this book will help you minimize resistance of all kinds in your swimming. You will even reduce the internal resistance caused by unwanted muscle tension or poor range of motion in joints, as you refine your stroke technique and improve your flexibility. Suffice it to say that the less resistance you work against, the more efficient you will be in the water. You will have greater control over your workout, look more proficient as a swimmer, have more fun, and feel better about doing it all again.

Training With Skill Drills

We have designed a conditioning program around drills and exercises that will allow you to practice excellent swimming skills in a graduated fashion, while conditioning the muscles and ranges of motion required to execute those skills repeatedly over long distances.

Following are a series of skill drills that teach your body what it feels like to be in the correct positions and go through the correct motions that will eventually be part of an efficient freestyle stroke. You will want to spend time on each drill before you begin doing full workouts. Do all these drills with easy kicking. I encourage you to wear flippers on any drill you have not yet mastered.

Balance

Our first few drills are called *balance drills.* They teach your body what it feels like to be balanced in the water. For all but the best swimmers, our sense of balance in water is not well developed. Partly because we haven't spent nearly as much time in the water as we have on land, and partly because the consequences of not being balanced in the water aren't as dire as they are on land. In fact, most people don't even know what it feels like to be truly balanced in the water.

What Does It Mean to Balance in the Water?

In general, a balanced position for freestyle is one in which the head, torso, hips, and legs are all in one line, parallel to the surface of the water. This position allows minimal frontal resistance, the largest of the resistance forces a swimmer encounters. The concept of balance is fundamental to efficient swimming.

Many swimmers understand the need to have their whole body parallel to the surface but do it the wrong way. They use a strong kick to lift the hips and legs to the surface. Kicking uses a tremendous amount of energy. Great swimmers use a different approach that requires little or no energy expenditure to achieve this balanced position. Here are some keys to achieving and maintaining balance while swimming.

- **Keep your head in line.** Weighing 12 to 16 pounds, your head and its position have a great influence on the balance of your body in the water. The crown of your head needs to be in line with your spine. Lifting your head off this line puts a large downward force on your hips, causing them to sink. You can easily feel this by lying face down on the ground, hands at your sides, and lifting your head straight up off the ground. You will feel your hips press toward the ground. The position of your head is critically important to maintaining a balanced position. When you are balanced, whether on your stomach, side, or back, only about one-quarter to one-third of your head will be exposed above the surface. The rest will be underwater.

- **Press your buoy.** Your lungs are literally a buoy that causes the upper portion of your body to float. By contrast, your center of mass, located near your belly button, causes your hips and legs to sink. Imagine a kickboard placed on the water's surface. If you press on one end of the kickboard, the other end rises. Pressing your buoy

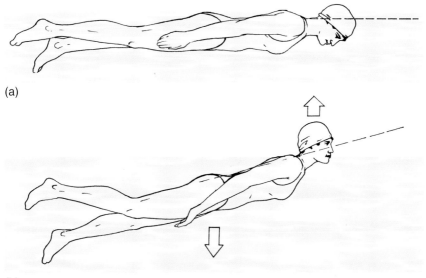

(a)

(b)

(a) Keeping the crown of your head in line with your spine will help you stay balanced. (b) Lifting your head off the spine line, even a little, will immediately and dramatically drive your hips toward the bottom of the pool, destroying balance. The dotted line on each figure depicts the spine line.

toward the bottom or leaning on it raises the hips in much the same
way that pressing on one end of the kickboard raises the other end.
The overall feeling you should get as you press your buoy is one of
tilting slightly downhill. I will review the concept of maintaining
balance by keeping your head in line and pressing your buoy toward
the bottom throughout this section.

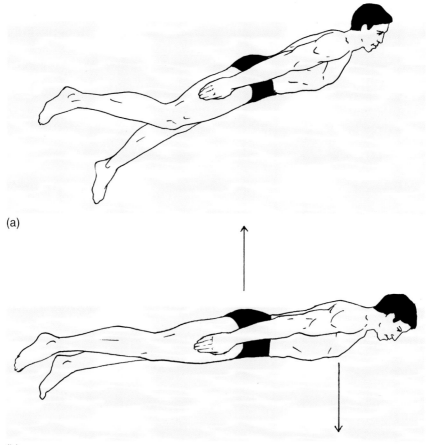

(a)

(b)

By putting pressure on your buoy, you will be properly streamlined in the water:
(a) Lean on your chest and feel your hips rise to the surface. (b) With the right
amount of pressure on your chest, you'll feel your entire body supported in a
balanced position.

The balance drills we use are divided into two groups: *static balance drills,*
which teach you what it feels like to be balanced in a variety of positions,
and *dynamic balance drills,* which teach you how to stay balanced as you
move from one position to another.

Static Balance Drills

As we move through the drills, I will introduce some terms and concepts with which you may be unfamiliar and will define or explain these at the end of the drill. Also, each drill will have one or more feedback points that will help you know if you are doing the drill correctly.

Front Balance (FB). Push off from the wall on your stomach, with both arms at your sides, and begin kicking easily. Keep your head in line; the crown of your head should be in line with your spine, nose pointed toward the bottom of the pool. Lightly press your buoy toward the bottom. This will raise your hips to the surface. When you need to take a breath, lift your head straight up in front and get a breath of air. Then put your head down so the crown is in line with your spine, and press your buoy again. When you lift your head, your hips and legs sink rapidly toward the bottom. Also, note that as soon as you get your head in line with your spine and press your buoy, you again get balanced.

FEEDBACK POINT The back quarter of your head, your shoulder blades, and the cheeks of your butt will be exposed to the air when you are in balance.

Back Balance (BB). Push off from the wall on your back, both arms at your sides, nose pointed up, breathing freely. Begin kicking easily. Lightly press your buoy (lean on a spot between your shoulder blades) toward the bottom.

FEEDBACK POINT When you are in balance, only about one-quarter of your head (i.e., just your face) will be exposed above the water surface. Your ears will be underwater, your pelvis should be within an inch of the surface, and your knees or feet should occasionally touch the surface as you continue kicking.

Side-Glide Balance (SGB). Push off from the wall on your side, with the lower arm extended straight toward the end of the pool, your other arm pressed lightly along your side, and your nose pointed up, breathing freely. Begin kicking easily. The back of your head should be in contact, or nearly in contact, with your extended arm. Stay in this side-lying, nose-up position for the length of the pool. Do this drill on both sides.

FEEDBACK POINT When you are balanced on your side, you will be able to feel a strip of flesh exposed to the air all the way down your side arm from shoulder to wrist. Putting more pressure on your buoy by leaning in on your armpit will help this. Your extended arm should feel weightless. Note that when you are balanced, your head should be in the same position as in the back balance drill—ears underwater, nose straight up, and only about a quarter of your head exposed to the air.

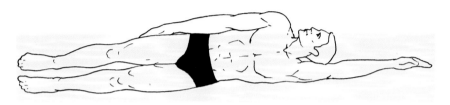

Side-glide balance drill.

Vertical Kicking (VK). Go to a section of the pool that is over your head in depth. As the name indicates, this is a kicking drill in a vertical position. Place one hand over the other on your chest and start kicking to hold your head at the surface, with the mouth and nose out of the water. Keep your back and head position straight up and down, resisting the temptation to lean forward. Kick mainly from the hips, allow your knees to yield slightly to the pressure of the water, and keep your ankles loose. Keep your kick small and rapid. Kick in this manner for 15 seconds and rest (hold the lane rope or side) for 15 seconds. Start with small doses of this drill, perhaps six repetitions of 15 seconds kick, followed by 15 seconds rest. After you gain confidence, add more repetitions. You can graduate the difficulty and training value of the drill by holding your hands just above the surface, on top of your head, or in full streamline position during the kicking.

Although vertical kicking is not technically a balance drill, it is an excellent drill to do early in your training. Most adult swimmers spend huge amounts of energy on kicking when swimming. There are several reasons for this: (1) They are using kicking to try to lift the butt and legs to the surface (you now know that pressing your buoy answers this problem); (2) they are displaying poor ankle flexibility (you now know that flippers are your answer here); or (3) the swimmer is kicking with incorrect leg motion—bicycle kicking or kicking mainly from the knees. Vertical kicking will cure incorrect kicking motions faster than anything I know. Survival instincts will allow your neuromuscular system to quickly figure out which motions are most effective in keeping your blowhole

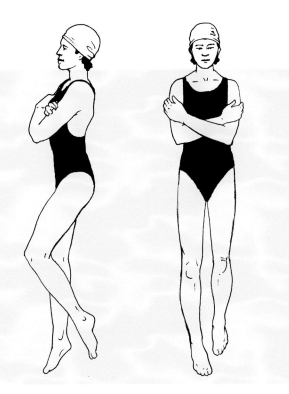

Vertical kicking drill.

exposed. If you find that this drill is impossible to survive as described, wear flippers for a few days, then begin to wean yourself from them.

Dynamic Balance Drills

The following drills will help you learn how to maintain balance while performing simple movements.

Side-Glide Balance With Breathing (SGBB).   Same drill as the side-glide balance drill but this time, after getting balanced and taking several breaths in the nose-up position, turn your head so your nose points toward the bottom of the pool, and exhale underwater. As you finish exhaling, turn your head again so you are in the nose-up position. Take several breaths in this position before doing another underwater exhalation. The only thing that moves in this drill is your head. The body should stay in the same balanced side-lying position throughout the drill. As you practice this drill, keep taking fewer breaths each time you turn your head to the nose-up position, until you turn your head only for a single breath. Do this drill on both sides.

FEEDBACK POINT When your nose points up, your head should be in the same position as in the side-glide balance drill—ears underwater. When your nose points toward the bottom, only the back quarter of your head should be exposed. The idea is to rotate your head as if it is on a skewer (through your crown and along your spine), without bending the skewer. Feel for that dry strip of flesh down your side arm, from shoulder to wrist, at all times in this drill. There is a tendency to lift the head when turning to the nose-up position. This results in the hips dropping, and you'll feel the waterline creep up your side arm toward your shoulder, indicating you have lost balance.

A common tendency on this drill is to allow the extended arm to fall toward the bottom as the head turns for the breath. This is the result of lifting the head slightly. The cure is to be aware of keeping the extended arm weightless and aiming straight toward the far wall. As you roll your body, press the side and back of your head lightly toward the bottom of the pool. Try to have contact, or at least very little daylight, between the back of your head and the extended arm. You can even think of lifting the extended arm slightly, perhaps one inch, toward the surface as you roll to breathe.

Balanced Body Rolling (BBR). Push off from the wall in the same position you used in the front balance drill, on your stomach with both arms at your sides, nose pointed toward the bottom of the pool, and begin kicking easily. Keep the crown of your head in line with your spine, and keep enough pressure on your buoy to stay balanced. When you need a breath, roll onto your back, keeping your hands at your sides and keeping pressure on your buoy as you roll. Begin rolling your body before you turn your head. If you roll your body before your head and keep pressure on your buoy as you roll, you will already be in a balanced position when you reach your back (the same position as in the back balance drill). Stay balanced while breathing freely on your back. After you are sure you are well balanced and have taken a couple breaths, roll again to your front. Begin rolling the body before turning the head, and keep pressure on your buoy as you roll. Do this drill rolling in both directions.

FEEDBACK POINT As you roll from the front position to the back position, you should feel the flesh from your shoulder to your wrist exposed to the air all at once, as you roll through the side position toward your back. The same is true when rolling from your back to your front. You may find you need more pressure on your buoy to stay balanced when on your side. There may be a strong tendency to turn the head first before rolling the body. This *always* results in lifting the head and destroying balance.

Stroke Integration

Our next drills are *stroke integration drills.* We will work with positions and motions that we used in the balance drills but add arm motions as we move from position to position. Stroke integration drills allow you to take discrete skills you have learned and integrate them into one coordinated set of motions that propels you easily and quickly down the pool. First, I want to explore a couple concepts important to proper stroke integration.

Swimming on Your Sides

As mentioned before, the water offers less resistance when we are in a side-lying position. This means we want to swim freestyle as much on our sides as possible and avoid spending time on our stomachs. An efficient freestyle stroke is a series of alternating right and left side-lying glides, connected by snappy rolls of the body from one side position to the next.

Swimming Engine Is in the Hips

As luck would have it, rolling from one side to the other allows the swimmer to involve much more muscle mass and power in the swimming effort than when swimming flat. Take the baseball pitcher who hurls 90 mile per hour fastballs over the plate. Where is most of the work being done? His legs, hips, and torso do most of the work. Freestyle swimming is no different. We want to use the rotation of the hips and torso as the predominant source of propulsive forces and allow our shoulders, arms, and hands to act more as transmissions than engines.

How can rotating the hips in a plane at right angles to our intended motion propel us toward the far wall? Let me venture into the home handyman's world for another analogy: the common screwdriver. Your hand applies a rotational force to the handle of the screwdriver. How is it that this rotational force causes the shaft of the screw to move linearly through the great resistance of a piece of wood? The threads on the screw shaft grip and hold onto a spot in the wood, effectively transmitting the rotational force applied at the handle into the linear motion of the screw shaft.

In swimming, when the hips begin to rotate, the trunk muscles stretch and twist around the spine. When these muscles contract, the combined large forces of hip and trunk rotation are transmitted through the shoulder and upper arm to the lower arm and hand. The job of the forearm and hand is, primarily, to find and hold onto a spot in the water, allowing the hip and trunk rotational forces to be applied linearly to the water, thus propelling the rotating shaft of the body through the great resistance of the water. The hands and arms serve roughly the same function in the water as the screw threads do in the piece of wood—to grip and hold onto one spot while the shaft rotates past that spot. Attempting to pull too hard or "move water" is analogous to stripping the threads on the screw. As soon as you do, the rotational forces are no longer being transmitted to the water and are therefore wasted.

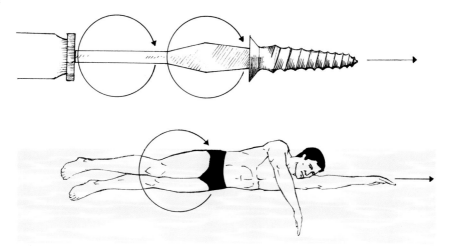

The threads on a screw lock into and hold a spot in the wood, allowing the rotational force that you apply to the screwdriver to be transmitted into linear motion through the great resistance of the wood. Likewise, the stroking arm and hand hold onto a spot in the water, allowing the rotational force applied at the hips to be transmitted into linear motion through the great resistance of the water.

Aside from making swimming more powerful and fluid, using body rotation to power our strokes has great fitness benefits. By using body rotation in this manner, we can involve up to five times as much muscle mass in our swimming motions as we would if swimming flat. When you exercise more muscle mass during a workout, you greatly magnify the fat-burning effects of increased metabolism during the next few hours.

Front Quadrant Swimming

In the 1840s it was discovered that the shape of a vessel in the water, and the ratios of length, width, and depth, determined the amount of wave drag that vessel would have at any given speed. This concept is responsible for racing boats of all kinds being long and sleek looking. The implication for swimming is that drag and the power required to overcome it are significantly reduced when the body is as long as possible and stays that way during each stroke cycle.

Imagine a sailing event in which two evenly matched racing boats and crews are pitted against one another. Also imagine that once every second one of the boats morphs into a tugboat shape for half a second, then morphs back to racing-boat shape. You know intuitively to bet on the other boat, because it keeps its long, sleek shape. I need to define some terminology here, before I liken swimmers to boats. I break a single-arm stroke cycle into three parts:

1. **The stroke.** The propulsive action of getting the hand from the fully extended position in front of the body, along a line straight down the center of the body, through the water to the finish position at the side of the body just past the hip. The stroke starts as the body begins to roll from one side-lying position and ends as the body finishes rolling to the other side-lying position.

2. **The recovery.** The nonpropulsive action of picking up and carrying the arm from just below the hip, through the air to a point where the hand is even with the top of the head. The body stays on its side while recovering—no rolling at all—just gliding.

3. **The entry.** The movement of the arm and hand from the point even with the top of the head to full extension. The entry starts as the body begins to roll from one side-lying position and ends as the body finishes rolling to the other side-lying position. To the casual observer, the arm should appear to enter and extend toward the far wall as a result of the body roll, rather than the hand stabbing forward from the shoulder. From here we go back to 1, the stroke, to start a new stroke cycle.

Note that the last sentence of the stroke definition and the second sentence of the entry definition are nearly identical. Also, because your arm motions are alternating, while the right arm is engaged in 1, the left arm is engaged in 3, and vice versa.

Now, let's take the average six-foot tall person who, when stretched to full streamline position, becomes an eight-foot six-inch to nine-foot long vessel in the water. Let's have him swim along at a moderate pace, being sure that he is getting into a fully streamlined, side-lying position on each stroke. We'll call this the racing-boat shape.

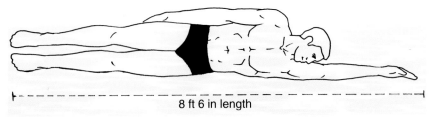

8 ft 6 in length

Racing-boat shape.

Now, say he begins his recovery and his stroke at the same time so his recovering arm and pulling arm are passing the shoulders at about the same time. We'll call this the tugboat shape. This swimmer alternately morphs from the racing-boat shape to the tugboat shape and back as he swims.

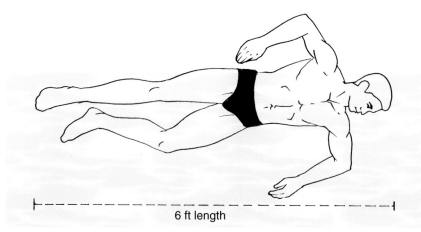

6 ft length

Tugboat shape.

Now the woman in the next lane (same height, same racing-boat shape) has figured out how to keep from morphing into the tugboat shape. Instead of starting her recovery and pull together, she begins and completes her recovery before she begins her arm stroke. In this way she maintains her streamlined, side-lying position, and most of it's length, for nearly the entire stroke cycle. Then, there is a rapid transition of the hips and body from one side to the other as the recovering hand enters the water and the stroking arm begins to do its thing.

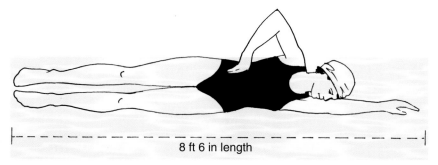

8 ft 6 in length

Still a racing-boat shape.

This is called *front quadrant swimming*. The large circle in the following figure shows that the recovering hand of the woman is about to enter the water while her stroking hand is still in the front quadrant. Another way of thinking about this is to be aware of where your hands pass each other as your recovering hand moves forward to enter the water and your working or stroking hand moves in the opposite direction. Your passing zone should be at, or forward of, your head.

Staying on your side and keeping an arm outstretched in front of the body at all, or most, times during the stroke allows the average length of

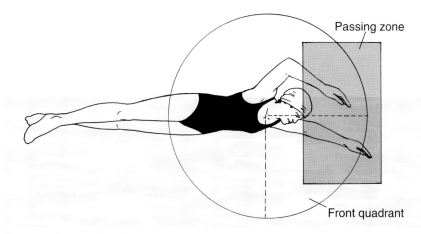

Front quadrant swimming.

the vessel in the water to stay long, thus reducing wave drag dramatically. These stroke integration drills will reinforce this.

Stroke Integration Drills

So, how do we get all these concepts—swimming on your sides, using body rotation as your primary propulsion source, and front quadrant swimming—integrated into normal swimming? Just as we use drills to teach the body the concepts of static balance and dynamic balance, we'll now introduce you to several more complex drills to tie this into swimming strokes. Before you go to the stroke-integration drills, though, you should have practiced all the balance drills until they are comfortable to you.

Side-Front-Side (SFS). Push off from the wall on your side with the lower arm extended straight toward the end of the pool, your other arm pressed lightly along your side, and your nose pointed down (same as in the side-glide balance drill except the nose position. Keep pressure on your buoy to stay balanced. Begin kicking easily. Recover your side arm over the surface of the water, and roll your body to the front position while sliding your recovering hand forward to enter the water and contact the back of the extended hand (see *The Glove* on p. 45). Stop rolling but continue kicking in the front position for a three-count, both arms extended, to be sure you are balanced. Then continue the roll, allowing your head to turn with the body and stroking the other arm down the centerline of the body. Roll and stroke such that you reach the opposite side-lying position at the same instant you finish the stroke. As you reach the side-lying position, continue turning your head so your nose is pointed nearly straight up. Continue kicking in this side-lying, nose-up position long enough to double-check your side balance feedback points, breathing freely and making corrections if necessary. Once you are sure you are balanced, turn your nose back

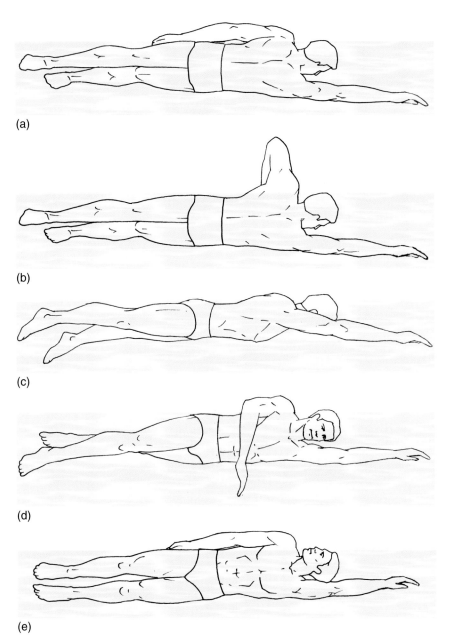

(a)

(b)

(c)

(d)

(e)

Side-front-side drill (a) nose-down side glide; (b) midrecovery; (c) front, arms extended; (d) midstroke; and (e) nose-up side glide.

toward the bottom and continue kicking on your side for 10 kicks or more. You are now in the same position on the side opposite the one you started on. Repeat these actions for each arm in turn for the length of the pool.

Be patient with the side-front-side drill. This is the drill in which your brain and body want to rush things and try to get into the next stroke right away. Resist this temptation. As you get better at doing the side-front-side drill you will gain confidence in your ability to remain balanced as you roll. You will know this once you seldom or never need to make balance corrections after reaching either the front position or your side position before breathing.

FEEDBACK POINT For balance on your side, feel for a dry strip of flesh from shoulder to wrist. Keep your extended arm weightless. As you roll to the front position, be sure to keep pressure on your buoy so you feel the front balance feedback points—back of your head, shoulder blades, and butt cheeks—exposed at the surface. As you roll onto your other side, keep pressure on your buoy so your hips stay at the surface and you expose your flank to the air. It is important that your head and body roll from the front position as a unit rather than head first. Think, head and butt move together. When you reach the nose-up position, the back of your head should contact or nearly contact your extended arm.

Mental Image: The Glove. Among other things, the side-front-side drill exaggerates the concept of front quadrant swimming explained earlier. Most novice and intermediate swimmers are rear quadrant swimmers. To make the change to front quadrant swimming, it is useful to exaggerate it while doing drill work. During this drill, I encourage swimmers to imagine that the extended hand has a loose-fitting glove on it. Slide the recovering hand along the top of the extended hand into the glove. As soon as the fingertips of the recovering hand slip under the cuff of the glove, the palm of the glove opens, allowing the extended arm to start stroking while the recovering hand continues to slide forward into the glove. The idea is to keep transferring the glove from hand to hand in this manner. Keep in mind that when swimming instead of drilling, we will not actually have contact between the two hands in front of the body. We do, however, want the recovering arm to nearly catch up to the extended arm before the extended arm takes the next stroke.

Side-Glide Freestyle (SGF). This drill is a variation of the side-front-side drill. In the side-glide freestyle drill, we eliminate the stop in the front position and the stop in the nose-up position. Push off from the wall and begin kicking in the same balanced side-glide position, nose down. Recover your side arm over the surface of the water. As the recovering hand passes the head, begin to roll your body while sliding your recovering hand forward to enter the water. Instead of stopping in the front position, continue rolling through the front position to the other side-lying position, allowing your head to turn with the body and stroking the other arm down the centerline of the body. As before, roll and stroke so the stroke and roll finish at the same time, turning your head to the nose-up position. Now, instead of pausing in the nose-up position, take a breath, turn your nose toward the bottom, and continue kicking on your side for 10 kicks or more. You are now in the same position on the side opposite the one you started on. Repeat these actions for each arm in turn for the length of the pool.

As you continue to make progress with this drill, gradually decrease the amount of kicking you do in each side-glide position. Also, practice side-glide freestyle with different breathing patterns. As you get comfortable with this drill, take some strokes without turning your head to breathe, remaining nose down. Breathing every second or third stroke are common breathing patterns.

FEEDBACK POINT When on your side, feel for a dry strip of flesh from shoulder to wrist. Keep your extended arm weightless. Keep pressure on your buoy as you roll, so your hips stay at the surface through the front position and onto your other side, exposing your flank to the air. Feel for your head and hips to rotate together to breathe.

Three and Glide (3&G). This drill is halfway between drilling and swimming, calling for you to take three strokes and pause in the side-glide position. Start by pushing off the wall and kicking in the side-glide position on your right side, nose down. As soon as you are well balanced, recover the trailing (left) arm over the water, roll, and stroke onto your left side as you did in the side-glide freestyle drill, except keep your head in the nose-down position. Now begin immediately to recover the trailing (right) arm; then roll and take the second stroke onto your right side. As soon as you get back to your right side, recover the trailing (left) arm, roll, and take your third stroke onto the left side. As you get fully onto your side, stop all action except kicking and spend several seconds in the side-glide position to assess and correct balance. Note that you are now gliding on the opposite side from which you started. After you are fully relaxed and balanced, turn your face to the nose-up position, grab a breath (or two if need be), turn your face back to the nose-down position, and assess and correct balance. Next, go through another set of three strokes to get to your original side-glide position on your right side. Kick along on that side for a few seconds, turn your head to breathe, turn it back to nose down, and check and correct balance. Repeat the entire process until you reach the other end of the pool.

When you first try the three and glide drill, breathe only while you are in side-glide position between sets of three strokes. If you need to, take several breaths while in this position. After you have mastered this drill, you may switch to breathing on the first or second stroke of each cycle of three strokes. Be sure to allow your head to roll along with the body roll to get air, as you did in the side-glide freestyle drill.

FEEDBACK POINT Each time you roll and stroke, be aware of your belly button pointing directly toward the side wall, as it is when in side-glide position. Each time you take a stroke, be sure you are swapping hands in front of the body, perhaps using *The Glove* from time to time. As you finish the third stroke of each set and hold the side-glide position, you want to immediately feel the dry strip of flesh down your trailing arm. If not, this tells you that you lifted your head up, let pressure off your buoy, or both.

As you get better at the three and glide drill, you can take more strokes in each set of strokes, effectively turning this into the five and glide or seven and glide drill. Increase the number of strokes only when you can enter each glide phase in a fully balanced position that needs no correction.

Fine Tuning Stroke Integration

As I stated earlier, swimming is the most complex set of repetitive motions in sport. The drills we've covered will have a more beneficial effect on your swimming than anything else I could mention. However, after you've mastered those drills you may find yourself searching for more things to keep your gray matter active. Following are a few more focus points you can employ in your drilling and in your swimming.

Focus Point: Marionette High Elbow Recovery. Until now, I haven't said much about how to recover your arm; allow me to correct that now. Imagine you are a marionette. Your puppeteer has only one string attached—to the elbow on your recovering arm. Assuming you are in the side-glide position, the puppeteer lifts your arm out of the water by tugging on that string. Your elbow goes straight up while your forearm and hand hang down relaxed from the elbow, with the fingertips near the water surface (perhaps even dragging on the surface) and staying in close to the body. As the elbow travels toward the front of the body, the hand follows a nearly straight line forward to the entry point, never straying far from the body or the water surface. Just as the elbow goes past the head, the string breaks and the whole arm structure topples forward into the water, with the recovering hand headed toward your extended hand.

Focus Point: Laser Beam Body-Roll Trigger. I've talked about what the side-glide positions look like and rolling from one side position to the other, but I haven't said much about when to roll. Assuming you have tried the marionette high elbow recovery, let me add another visual image.

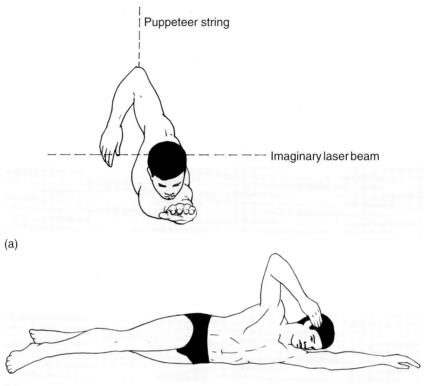

| Puppeteer string

— — — — — — — — — — — — — — — — — — Imaginary laser beam

(a)

(b)

Marionette high elbow recovery drill (a) head-on view of swimmer in side-lying position and (b) side view in which we can see the recovering hand passing the ear.

Imagine there is a laser beam stretching across your lane at the front edge of your head, approximately six inches higher than the water surface. As your puppeteer lifts your elbow by the string, you should stay on your side with your other hand fully extended. As the elbow, forearm, and hand move forward, nothing else should change (i.e., you *stay* on your side and *keep* the other hand fully extended). When the recovering hand cuts through the laser beam, this should be the trigger to begin rolling (in the side view of the marionette high elbow recovery figure, the recovering hand is about to cut this imaginary laser beam). As you begin to roll, the recovering hand continues forward, through the surface of the water to full extension, while the extended arm begins to take a stroke. Using this visual image will result in a near-perfect front quadrant stroke.

Focus Point: Hip Snap Power Surge. So, through all this drill stuff you've been thinking to yourself, "OK Coach, you're giving me lots of detail about balance, reducing resistance, gliding, and all that other efficiency stuff, but now I want to know how to go *faster!*" So, here I yield to your passion and divulge the secret of going faster: hips. Remember the screwdriver analogy? If you want that screw to go into the wood faster, you have to rotate the screwdriver faster. If you want your body to move faster, you have to rotate your hips faster. The faster you get from one side-lying position to the other side-lying position, the faster your stroking arm gets from the fully extended position in front to the finish position past your hip. Don't confuse this with trying to get to the next stroke quickly. In fact, the stronger a stroke is (i.e., the faster you snap your hips from one side to the other), the faster you will be going and the farther you can glide in the side position. So hip snap power surge is a way to focus on where your power comes from. Try it with any drill involving roll that you feel comfortable with and don't need 100-percent concentration to execute well. Think about starting the roll from your hips, and see how quickly you can get from your belly button facing one side wall to facing the other side wall.

Focus Point: Vertical Forearm Stroke.   If you have read much about swimming technique, you probably have been inundated with information about what the hands and arms do during the propulsive stroke portion of the arm cycle. *The fact is that how you take a stroke is not nearly as important as what you do while you are not stroking.*

However, some people would not feel that they had gotten their money's worth if I didn't address what the hand and arm do during the underwater part of the stroke. Here it is: Get the stroking forearm vertical to the pool bottom as far out in front of you as possible, and keep it vertical as long as possible while the arm moves down the length of the body. Note that the elbow is higher than an imaginary line between the wrist and the shoulder. This is referred to as swimming with a high elbow.

A common problem swimmers have is called the *dropped elbow,* which causes the forearm to be horizontal or near horizontal, minimizing the surface area available to hold onto the water. Swimming with a dropped elbow, the stroke creates lots of turbulence and little propulsion.

When swimming, concentrate on achieving the vertical forearm position as far in front of the body as possible. This may feel somewhat like rolling your hand and arm over a barrel or it may feel as though you are trying to run your elbow up over your hand before stroking. As you move the arm through the stroke, concentrate on keeping the forearm vertical as long as possible. Keeping the forearm vertical lets you hold onto a spot in the water speed without slipping water, thus allowing continuous transmission of body roll forces to the water for propulsion.

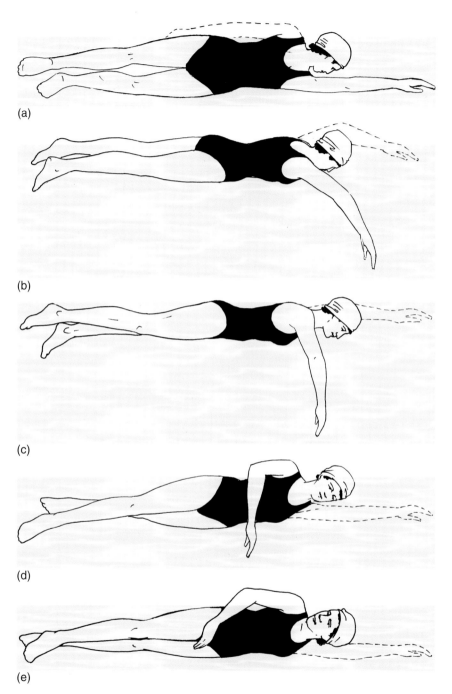

(a)

(b)

(c)

(d)

(e)

The vertical or nearly vertical forearm of the dotted arm allows you to use a maximum surface area—the entire forearm and hand—to hold onto a spot in the water.

Turning

Whether swimming or drilling, once you get to the wall you need to do one of two things: turn or get out. Assuming you opt for the former, there are a few considerations. What you want to accomplish with any turn is rapidly transitioning the body position from moving in one direction to moving in the opposite direction, in a minimum time, without losing speed, using the smallest amount of energy possible.

You could do a flip turn, that somersault-looking thing the fast swimmers do when they swim freestyle, or you can do an open turn, the turn used for breaststroke and butterfly. The open turn allows you to take a breath at the wall, but the flip turn does not. For just a lap or two this isn't a big deal. However, for distances of 200 yards or more, this difference adds up. For triathletes who need to be able to hop, skip, and jump out of the water; apply a flurry of activity in the transition area; and speed away on that ridiculously expensive two-wheeled toy, this one breath per length differential has far-ranging consequences. Finally, flip turns are far more complex and take much longer to learn than open turns. So, if vanity has you still desperately wanting to do flip turns, go see your local swim coach. However, a lightning-fast open turn as described below will be faster than 80 percent of the flip turns you are likely to encounter.

Open Turns. As you near the end of the pool, take your last stroke aggressively, making sure you get fully into your balanced side-glide position with one arm extended in front of you, your belly button facing the side wall, and the trailing arm just at the surface of the water. Execute the entire turn and push-off with your belly button facing the side wall. Keep kicking as you finish this last stroke and until your extended hand touches the wall, open and flat. Bend the wall arm slightly as your swimming momentum continues to move your body toward the wall. Avoid grabbing the gutter. Draw your legs up tightly under you, and swing your hips toward the wall as you push your upper torso away from the wall with your arm. Leave your trailing arm near the surface rather than moving it with your hips. The momentum of your body is what swings your hips toward the wall, as your body pivots around a point in your midsection.

As the wall arm pushes off the wall, your torso is straight up and down with your legs tucked in tight under you in midswing toward the wall. Your hand then swings straight over your head, as your whole body continues to pivot. At this instant, no part of your body contacts the wall.

As your body continues to pivot, untuck your legs and keep arcing the arm straight over your head. As your upper torso pivots down into the water, you want the top arm to meet the trailing arm below the surface of the water at the same instant your feet contact the wall—just toes and balls, not flat-footed. Place one hand and wrist on top of the other hand and

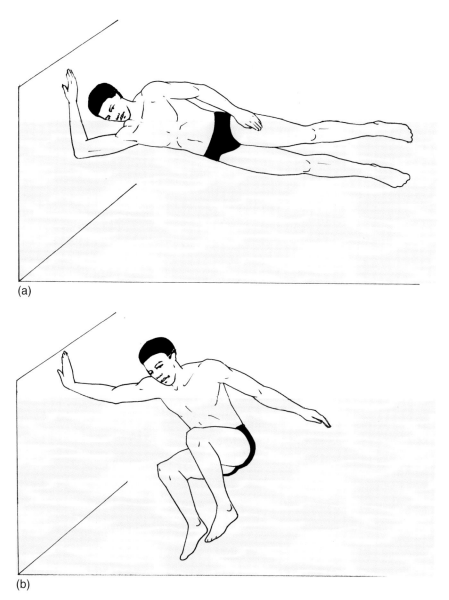

(a)

(b)

Open turn (a) wall contact, bent arm; (b) arm pushing off from wall, legs swinging up; (c) hand coming over head, feet nearing wall; and (d) feet pushing off wall.

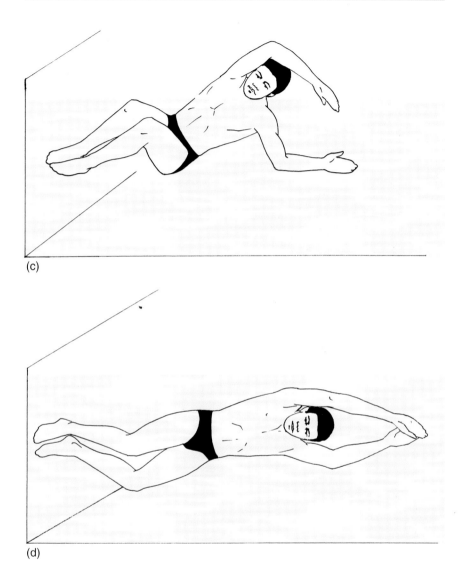

(c)

(d)

wrist, locking the thumb of the top hand around the edge of the bottom hand. All your fingers should point straight toward the other end of the pool. Your torso should be fully submerged—12 to 18 inches below the surface of the water. The instant your feet touch the wall, explosively launch yourself off the wall as you snap into a fully streamlined glide position. Your goal is to allow your feet to languish on the wall no longer than a bouncing golf ball stays on the ground.

As you leave the wall, you want your body as long and narrow as possible—like an arrow—both arms extended toward the far wall. Squeeze your ears firmly between your upper arms, and point your toes toward the wall you just left. Finally, contract your abdominal muscles as though you are trying to press the small of your back against an imaginary wall. Your belly button is still facing the side wall. The line you push off on should be parallel with the surface, but 12 to 18 inches below the surface, to avoid gliding through the wave and surface turbulence that follows your body into the wall.

You travel faster in the first five yards after pushing off the wall than you will at any other point in the length—30- to 40-percent faster. Milk that push-off for everything it's worth with a streamlined glide; think of it as free speed. As you slow to swimming speed, begin a compact, rapid kick and, because you are still on your side, take your first stroke with the arm closest to the bottom of the pool so you can capitalize on body roll.

As you follow and practice the drills in the order presented in this chapter, you are, in effect, progressively building a new freestyle stroke from scratch. For a while, when you swim rather than practice drills, you will tend to revert to whatever stroke style you had before you read this book. However, the more comfortable and relaxed you become with these skills and drills, the easier they will be to incorporate into your everyday swimming. The workouts in subsequent chapters are built around progressively practicing the skill drills while first mixing in small, and later, larger amounts of full-stroke swimming.

Lap Swimming Etiquette

Whether it is an organized workout or a crowded lap swim session, you are likely to be sharing lane space with others from time to time. Everyone's water time is more enjoyable when we all know and live by the basic rules of swimming etiquette.

- **Read the signs.** Some pools post signs with the local version of swimming etiquette. If this is the case at your pool, follow the posted rules. Other signs may give some indications of how to fit in, such as posted speeds for lanes, direction of circle patterns, and so on.

- **Selecting and entering a lane.** Look for a lane with swimmers of your speed. Before entering a lane, communicate with the others in the lane so they know you are about to join them. If they are swimming nonstop, slip feet first (never dive into a lane with people swimming in it) into the right-hand corner of the lane and stay there long enough for everyone to cycle through the lane and see that a new swimmer has joined the fray. If, after a while, you find that you are frequently either passing people or being passed, you probably belong in another lane.

- **Circle pattern.** For any lane with more than two people swimming, all swimmers must swim in a circle pattern to avoid head-on collisions. This means that each swimmer swims down one side of the lane and back on the other side. Just like on the road, you should always stay to the right of your lane (unless otherwise posted). Each swimmer should leave at least a 5-second gap between him or herself and the next swimmer.

- **Drafting.** Just like in cycling, swimming close behind somebody allows you to benefit from the flow of water created by the lead swimmer. Although it may be tempting to tuck in behind someone and let them do most of the work, it is considered bad etiquette.

- **Passing and being passed.** Even in well-matched lanes, passing or getting passed is sometimes unavoidable when circle swimming. In general, the person passing should move to the center of the lane and speed up to finish the pass quickly. Likewise, the slower swimmer should anticipate being passed, stay close to the lane rope, and slow a bit to let the faster swimmer pass quickly. Alternatively, if you know you are about to be passed, you could stop briefly at the wall, allowing the faster swimmer to turn and take the lead. If you feel a tap on your foot, assume someone wants to pass you and act accordingly.

- **At the wall.** Regardless of how many swimmers are using a lane, it is everyone's responsibility to keep the center third of the wall at the end of the lane clear for other swimmers to turn. When you stop at the wall, move quickly to the far corner of the lane.

- **Do unto others.** Treat your lane partners with the same respect you would like to be treated with, and expect the same from them. Even a crowded lane can be a joy when everyone has that attitude.

5

Warming Up, Stretching, and Cooling Down

Visit nearly any pool at the appointed hour for a group workout and you will likely witness most of the group spending several minutes on deck before entering the water, going through motions and positions that might lead the unenlightened to assume they were all serious about stretching for flexibility. Add to this the fact that the coach must make several, progressively intense, exhortations for people to get in the water. The group appears united in their ardor for flexibility enhancement. The unenlightened are impressed by such a display. We coaches, on the other hand, are not.

You see, water that is the correct temperature for staying comfortably cool during a workout is usually uncomfortably cool when you first get in (the swimmers might call it shockingly cool while the coach refers to it as refreshingly cool). These few minutes (or perhaps much more if pressure is not brought to bear) of stretching are just an attempt to forestall the inevitable initial plunge with its few seconds of heart-stopping, lung-gripping semipanic that only grudgingly gives way to relative comfort after a few laps or more.

Real stretching is best done after you have warmed up or after you have completed your workout. Stretching should not be confused with warm-up. They are different activities with different goals and should happen at different times.

How to Warm Up

The best way to warm up is to get into the water and start swimming *slowly* for several laps. Immediately we are presented with a problem—if the water is cold you will likely have the inclination to sprint the first couple lengths to get your body temperature up. This can be a mistake. Better to know what temperature of water makes this initial sprint irresistible and take evasive action. In this event, it is best to do a dryland warm-up before chipping through the surface ice—calisthenics, a brisk walk, a bit of a jog, or whatever gets your body temperature up and your metabolism going. A good rule of thumb is your dryland warm-up should get you moderately sweaty. You want to hit the water immediately after your dryland warm-up, before you have a chance to cool down.

After your first couple laps adjusting to the water temperature, start getting your brain focused and your neuromuscular system correctly aimed. The progression of swimming skill drills detailed in chapter 4 makes an ideal warm-up regimen. Start with one length each of the static balance drills, then the dynamic balance drills, and finally the stroke integration drills. Spending an extra length or two on the drills that are harder for you to execute correctly is warranted here.

Using the skill drills as your warm-up forces your swimming muscles to go through all the ranges of motion required in full-stroke swimming but allows enough isolation of specific skills that you can easily focus on proper execution. Your brain

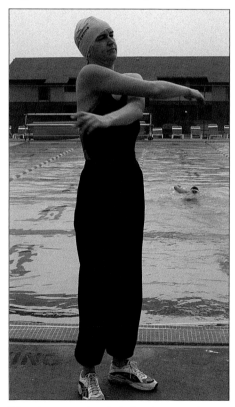

Warming up not only helps to prevent injury, it can also greatly improve performance by getting your body ready to work.

takes a while to get fully involved, and skill drills accomplish this effectively. Avoid the tendency to just do garbage yardage for your warm-up—only the foolish and the ignorant waste their time in this manner.

After you have gone through a set of skill drills, it's OK to do several laps of full-stroke swimming. Better yet, alternating a length of drill with a length of swim (focusing on making what you executed impeccably in your drill show up in your stroke) is an ideal way to work into full-stroke swimming. Plan on spending 10 to 15 minutes on your active in-water warm-up.

Stretching for Swimming

Stretching is about increasing range of motion (ROM). A variety of stretches are beneficial to swimmers, some more than others. Stretching is like broccoli—everyone knows it's good for you but few have a passion for it.

When to Stretch

You can choose to do your stretching during the workout or after. I prefer my swimmers to do a complete warm-up; then we do the two primary stretches noted in the following section. I also encourage them to do other stretching after the workout, but like broccoli, those often get slipped to the dog under the table.

How to Stretch

How you stretch is just as important as when you stretch and what stretches you do. To stretch safely and effectively, keep these rules in mind:

1. Move into each stretch position slowly, and stretch only to the point of mild discomfort.
2. Hold stretch positions steady for 20 to 30 seconds—never bounce.
3. Move out of the stretch position slowly.
4. Don't hold your breath during a stretch.

What Stretches to Do

There are two stretches I consider of paramount importance to swimmers. If you do no other stretches, do these. They are shown as you might do them in a pool because you should do them *every* time you get wet. You can also do them on land.

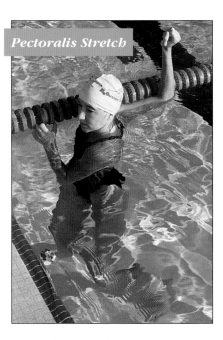

Stand in armpit deep water with your chest against the lane rope. Raise your right arm so that your upper arm is parallel with and alongside of the lane rope, with a 90-degree bend at the elbow so your fingertips are pointing straight up. Now rotate your body to the left. The lane rope keeps the arm from moving. As you rotate your body to the left, you should feel a stretch diagonally from the shoulder across your right pectoralis to the sternum (breast bone). If you just feel the stretch in the shoulder area, you need to raise your elbow higher until you feel the stretch across to the sternum. Otherwise, you aren't stretching the pectoralis muscle, you are just pulling the shoulder out of place. Repeat this stretch several times, alternating sides for 20 to 30 seconds each.

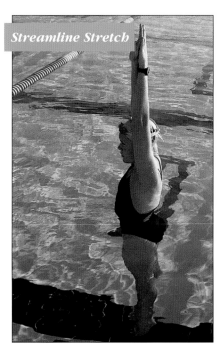

Stand up straight with both hands extended overhead as high as possible. Place your right hand over the left, locking your left thumb around the edge of your right hand. All your fingers should be pointing straight up. Your right wrist should be directly on top of your left wrist. Now squeeze your ears firmly between your upper arms. Stand up on your toes. Squeeze your butt cheeks together. Finally, contract your abdominal muscles as though you are trying to press the small of your back against an imaginary wall. This stretch is great for extending the range of shoulder motion needed for swimming as well as stretching your back for a streamlined glide position. Do this stretch at least twice for 20 to 30 seconds each time.

Other Stretches.   Other stretches that are useful to swimming include the following:

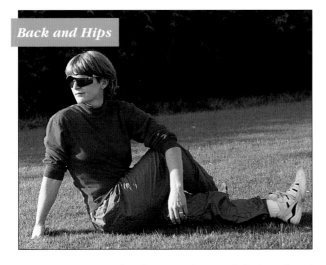

Back and Hips

Sit with your legs straight in front of you. Bend your right leg, cross it over your left knee, and place the sole of your right foot flat on the floor. Next, push against the outside of your upper right thigh with your left el-bow, just above the knee. Place your right hand behind you; then slowly rotate your upper body toward your right hand and arm. You should feel the stretch in your upper and lower back, hips, and buttocks.

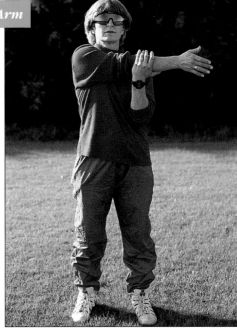

Upper Back, Shoulder, and Arm

With your left hand, grasp your right elbow and pull it slowly across your chest to-ward your left shoulder. You will feel the stretch along the outside of your right shoulder and arm. Repeat with the other arm.

Shoulders and Triceps

Bring both arms overhead and hold your left elbow with your right hand. Bend your left arm at the elbow and let your left hand rest against the right shoulder. Pull with your right hand to slowly move the left elbow behind your head until you feel a stretch. Repeat with the other arm.

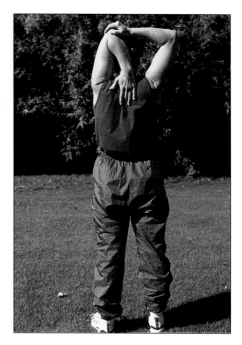

Ankle and Toe-Point Stretch

Sit on the floor with your knees bent so the bottoms of your feet are flat on the floor, facing your sofa (or any other object you can wedge your foot under). Wedge your right foot under it. Now, scoot back, straightening your right leg until you feel your ankle stretching. Scoot back only until you feel moderate discomfort. Hold this position for two or three minutes. Repeat with the other foot.

Cooling Down

Cooling down is like warming up in reverse. The idea is to slowly return the body and all its functions to near-resting levels over time by doing some easy swimming after your last hard effort. Ever hang around and listen to your car after you've turned it off following a long, hard drive—all those protesting sounds of metal ticking and vapor passing that go on for the next 10 minutes or so? Your body is the same. It protests when you swim it hard and put it up wet. The older the car is, the louder those protesting sounds are. Continued activity at a lower intensity—cooling down—avoids extra strain on the heart, and lessens postexercise cramping and soreness.

Use Cool-Down Effectively

People often think of cool-down time as garbage yardage because of the common misconception that you aren't getting any training effect while swimming at low intensity. Ignorance is bliss.

At the risk of waxing pedantic, I must stress again that the most important training you do in swimming is training your neuromuscular system (i.e., doing it *right* rather than just doing it). Cool-down is an excellent time to do some high-quality drill work. In fact, mentally coaxing your muscles to go through specific skill drills when they are fatigued presents an effective motor-learning opportunity. Choose drills you have mastered for cool-downs rather than ones you have difficulty executing.

PART II

SWIMMING WORKOUT ZONES

This part of the book uses six color-coded workout zones, arranged according to duration and intensity. Moving from one color to the next increases the intensity or the duration of the workout, but not both at the same time. Within each zone, there are 10 practices arranged in order of increasing difficulty.

Perceived Exertion

Heart rates are one way to quantify the intensity of a practice. Another way is to apply a rating of perceived exertion (RPE) developed by Dr. Gunnar Borg. On this subjective 10-point scale, 0 is the feeling of no exertion at all, 1 is very light, 2 is light, 3 is moderate, 4 is somewhat heavy, 5 is heavy, 7 is very heavy, and 10 is very, very heavy to maximum.

WORKOUT COLOR ZONES				
Zone (chapter)	Type of workout	RPE*	Target HR range	Duration
Green (6)	Low intensity, short duration	1-4	60-70%	20-30 min
Blue (7)	Low intensity, long duration	1-4	60-70%	30-40 min
Purple (8)	Medium intensity, short duration	4-7	70-85%	30-40 min
Yellow (9)	Medium intensity, long duration	4-7	70-85%	40-50 min
Orange (10)	High intensity, short duration	7-10	75-100%	40-50 min
Red (11)	High intensity, long duration	7-10	75-100%	50-60 min

*Rating of perceived exertion.

Measuring Your Heart Rates During Practices

Part of the conditioning methodology expressed here is based on monitoring your exercise heart rate regularly during practices. You will often see the acronym IHR (immediate heart rate) in the practice notation, asking you to check your working heart rate. There are several ways to vary the degree of difficulty from practice to practice within a zone:

1. Skill and drill complexity
2. Length of swims or sets of swims
3. Amount of rest
4. Intensity of swimming
5. Target heart rate range
6. Duration of the practice session

IHR (Immediate Heart Rate)

IHR is your heart rate taken immediately after an exertion. If you have an electronic heart rate monitor, use the first stable reading you get. To take a manual heart rate, use two fingers to locate your carotid artery just below the hinge point of your jaw, an inch or so below your earlobe, and feel your pulse. Count the number of beats you feel in 10 seconds. As you watch a clock, count 0 on the first beat that happens on or after any 5-second mark, then continue counting beats to and including the first beat that falls on or after the 10th second. (In the previous example, you finish on 10:30. You quickly locate your pulse. This takes you until the :37 mark.

On the :40, begin counting on the first beat you feel. Start with 0. Count all beats up to and including the first beat you feel on or after :50 mark.) Let's say you counted 25 beats. Multiply this number by six and you have your approximate heart rate of 150. If you are new to taking your heart rate in this manner, you will want to practice a few times. If you can do it sitting in your chair, you'll find it easier to do after physical exertion because the pulse beats will be easier to feel. Following is a heart rate conversion table.

Heart Rate Conversion Table	
10-second count heart rate	
15	90
16	96
17	102
18	108
19	114
20	120
21	126
22	132
23	138
24	144
25	150
26	156
27	162
28	168
29	174
30	180
31	186
32	192
33	198

Alternatively, you can count your heartbeats (just as you did previously) for six seconds and simply add a zero (i.e., if you count 14 heartbeats in six seconds your IHR is 140). Though simpler than counting for 10 seconds and multiplying by six, this method is less accurate.

Your General Aerobic Target Heart Rate Range

Before commencing any aerobic exercise regimen, you should know what range of heart rates is appropriate for you. This is referred to as your general aerobic target heart rate range (GATHRR). As long as you keep your heart rate in this range for at least 20 minutes, you can be sure of aerobic benefits from your practice. Follow these easy steps to find your GATHRR:

Step 1. Find your true resting heart rate (RHR). It is best to do this first thing in the morning before the alarm goes off. Alternatively, you could take your RHR after lying still for 20 to 30 minutes and at least 4 hours after consuming caffeine. Sunday afternoon naps are excellent for this. Count the number of pulses over a full 60-second period. Breathe normally while you are taking your RHR. Ideally, you should do this for several days and take the average.

Step 2. Estimate your maximum heart rate (MHR).

$$MHR = 220 - \text{your age}$$

Step 3. Figure your heart rate reserve (HRR)—the difference between your maximum heart rate and your resting heart rate.

$$HRR = MHR - RHR$$

Step 4. Figure your general aerobic target heart rate range (GATHRR).

The lower end of your GATHRR = (55% $\times$ HRR) + RHR $-$ 10
The upper end of your GATHRR = (85% $\times$ HRR) + RHR $-$ 10

(We subtract 10 beats per minute to adjust for the fact that heart rates react differently in the buoyant environment of the water than they do in the gravity-dominated land environment. This assumes that you take the heart rate in water up to your shoulders.)

Here's an example. Joe Swimmer is 35 years old with an RHR of 50.

$$MHR = 220 - 35 = 185$$
$$HRR = MHR - RHR = 185 - 50 = 135$$
Upper GATHRR = (.85 $\times$ HRR) + RHR $-$ 10 = (.85 $\times$ 135) + 50 $-$ 10 = 155
Lower GATHRR = (.55 $\times$ HRR) + RHR $-$ 10 = (.55 $\times$ 135) + 50 $-$ 10 = 114

His general aerobic training heart rate range is 114 to 155. When he takes 10-second IHRs, he will look for counts from 19 to 26. As long as he stays within this range while he is practicing, he can be sure he is getting aerobic benefit.

When your heart rate goes lower than your GATHRR, you are no longer getting aerobic benefit. When your heart rate goes higher than your GATHRR, the nature of the work is becoming more anaerobic. When you do your T-15, T-20, or T-30 swims, you should expect to finish with IHRs at or slightly higher than the upper end of your GATHRR. This is what is referred to as anaerobic threshold work—just at the threshold of anaerobic activity, the highest intensity of exercise that you can continue for an extended time. Research indicates that the fastest aerobic adaptations occur when you do work at this intensity.

Specific Target Heart Rate Ranges

Practices in each color zone have a suggested average effort level, expressed as a percentage range of maximum heart rate. This is your target heart rate range for most of the practice. Each practice has several places where you take an IHR. In general, your goal should be to attenuate your exertion level and gauge your rest periods so that your heart rate stays higher than the low end of the recommended target heart rate range. There will be some sets in many practices that will produce heart rates somewhat higher than this range. These heart rate peaks will be for short periods and will usually be accompanied by significant amounts of rest built into the practice, allowing your heart rate to return to within the specified target range. The higher you go in the color chart, the more often these peaks will occur—especially in the Orange and Red zones.

Caloric Cost

Good news for persons counting calories—sitting still and barely breathing burns calories. This is referred to as basal metabolism—the minimum number of calories we need to stay alive, even if we never got out of bed. Depending on age, body weight, amount of lean muscle mass, and general health, the number of calories burned per day varies from 1,800 to 3,000. Any activity we engage in after doing battle with the alarm clock adds to the total burned for the day.

Many people would like to know exactly how many calories they have burned at the end of a workout. Despite considerable research time and effort to accurately estimate caloric cost of exercise, we can give you only ranges within which your expenditure might fall.

Swimming is a particularly hard activity to assess caloric cost for. Ability level greatly affects total resistance the swimmer works against. A small person that swims ugly, thrashing water about and making waves while swimming slowly, likely burns more energy than a larger person swimming faster but with graceful, streamlined, efficient form. So body size, distance, and speed (a useful measure on land) won't do us much good for estimating caloric cost in swimming.

However, we can indirectly estimate caloric cost through heart rates. Although the speed and efficiency of the swimmer are directly reflected in the heart rate, there will still be some variance based on body size and conditioning level. The estimates here are for an average-size person, weighing 150 pounds, in average aerobic condition. Larger persons will burn more calories and smaller persons will burn fewer—add or subtract 15 percent for every 25-pound variance. Well-conditioned persons will burn more calories at any heart rate than less well-conditioned persons. There aren't long duration entries for the higher heart rates because it is not possible to do long bouts of exercise at near-maximal heart rates.

Calories Burned per Minute at Various MHR						
Percent of MHR	kcal/minute	20 min	30 min	40 min	50 min	60 min
55%	4	80	120	160	200	240
60%	5	100	150	200	250	300
65%	6	120	180	240	300	360
70%	7	140	210	280	350	420
75%	8	160	240	320	400	480
80%	9	180	270	360	450	540
85%	10	200	300	400	500	600
90%	11	220	330	440		
95%	12	240				
100%	13+					

Choosing Your First Training Zone

Start in the Green zone if (1) you scored under 10 points on the Swimming Fitness Test you took in chapter 3, (2) you are a NEBAB (never ever been athletic before), or (3) there are any skills or concepts in chapter 4 that are new to you. Chances are that you fall in one or more of these categories.

Because the Green zone consists primarily of body balance and swimming skill drills, these practices are also excellent for skill isolation and refinement for swimmers of any ability or conditioning level, or for a warm-up before more intense workouts. Regardless of swimming background, I encourage you to start in the Green zone and work through all the practices in the order presented. Skilled swimmers may find that they can breeze through more than one of these practices in a single pool session. Less skilled swimmers will likely do only one per pool session, and in fact may need to repeat a practice a couple times before moving to the next one.

If you start in an advanced zone, be sure to read through the information and practices for each of the prior zones to familiarize yourself with the terminology and training concepts presented.

When first starting with the workouts in this book, I strongly suggest that you go through the workouts in the Green through Yellow zones in the order presented. There is a logical order to the skills, drills, concepts, and work volume within each set of practices. If you find that you are struggling to complete workouts as you move through the section, it is advisable to backtrack, either returning to the beginning of the section or, perhaps, even to an earlier zone.

However, you should *not* approach the Orange and Red zones in this manner. Once you have gotten through the Yellow zone workouts, you should go on to one of the training programs in chapter 13. These two zones include too much high-intensity work to do them day after day.

Moving Up to the Next Training Zone

In any exercise regimen, there is a certain excitement, anticipation, and eagerness about moving up to the next level. However, for long-term success it is necessary to be fully prepared for each step up. Be sure to complete each practice in a zone before moving up to the next color. In the Green through Yellow zones, I encourage you to make at least two full passes through each color before trying the next color. You should be able to complete all the practices in a zone without straying out of the target training heart rate range for more than brief periods. You should also feel confident about all the skill drills and focus points presented in your current zone before moving up to the next color. If not, you may want to review and practice in the areas you are concerned about. Remember that when a skill eludes you, often the problem lies in having not mastered an earlier skill.

Once you have decided to move into the next color training zone, the practices will continually revisit the most fundamental skills. As the practices progress through the zone, a logical pattern of increasing skill difficulty will be apparent. This repeated cycling through all levels of skills is a cornerstone of your long-term stroke development.

Before you started on your swimming exercise program, you completed the T-15 swim (chapter 3, p. 24) and kept records of your performance. Each time you cycle through a set of practices in a zone, it is a good idea to repeat the T-15 swim and compare your new results with previous results. As you complete each zone, you should see some improvement in distance, speed, final heart rate, average stroke count, perceived exertion, or a combination of these. At some point you will feel confident about moving up to T-20 swims and eventually to T-30 swims. Certainly, by the time you have completed the Yellow, or fourth, zone you should be doing T-20s instead of T-15 swims.

Ability Levels Versus Conditioning Levels

In swimming, as with any sport, ability is a combination of technique and conditioning. In general terms, we can define ability as the intersection of three easy-to-measure factors: (1) How fast do you swim? (2) How long can you keep going? (3) How much energy do you consume while you do it?

It is common to confuse conditioning with ability or to discount the importance of technique, so ability and conditioning become synonymous in the athlete's eyes. For sports in which the motions are ones we are naturally suited for, like running, or the motions are closely constrained or controlled, like cycling, it is easy to blur the distinction between conditioning and ability. Technique in these sports is a much smaller component of overall ability than is conditioning. In sports such as golf or tennis, however, technique is a much larger component of ability than is conditioning.

Swimming falls in this latter category. Ability in swimming is 70- to 90-percent technique and only 10- to 30-percent conditioning. This explains what invariably happens when the 30-year-old, ex-college scholarship swimmer returns to the pool after more than 5 years of couch potatoing. Swimming at her totally-out-of-shape-so-I-gotta-go-real-easy-so-I-can-survive-this-workout pace, she still manages to swim circles around 75 percent of the swimmers in the pool, all of whom have been working out diligently for months or years. Her excellent technique, honed by years of refinement when she was swimming as a youth and in college, is still more or less intact. This allows her to start at a high level of ability, despite little or no conditioning.

The practices in part II put strong emphasis on improving technical ability, while also giving you a great conditioning workout. In the Green and Blue zones, 60 to 90 percent of each practice will be skill drills that isolate specific, critical aspects of great freestyle swimming. The remaining 10 to 40 percent are short (one or two lengths) swims with a specific concept or skill to focus on. As you move through the colors, there will be more emphasis on swimming. The Purple and Yellow zones will include 40- to 70-percent drills, and the Orange and Red zones will include 20- to 50-percent drills.

Each drill is abbreviated in the body of the workout. Following is a legend showing the full name of each drill abbreviation used throughout the workouts in part II, as well as the page in chapter 4 where the drill description appears. You may want to photocopy this and put it in a watertight sandwich bag to take poolside.

Drills Legend	
Abbreviation	**Drill**
FB	Front balance (p. 35)
BB	Back balance (p. 35)
SGB	Side-glide balance (p. 35)
SGBB	Side-glide balance with breathing (p. 37)
BBR	Balanced body rolling (p. 38)
SFS	Side-front-side (p. 43)
SGF	Side-glide freestyle (p. 45)
3&G	Three and glide (p. 46)
5&G	Five and glide (p. 47)
VK	Vertical kicking (p. 36)

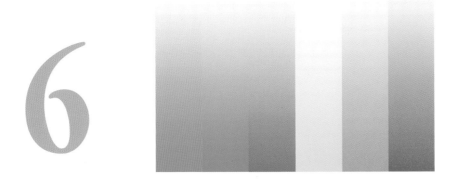

6

Green Zone

Workouts in the Green zone consist primarily of body balance and swimming skill drills with a small amount of full-stroke swimming. You may do them entirely with full-size or short-blade training fins. If you make good forward progress when kicking without fins, you can also do these workouts with naked feet. Assuming you start with full-size fins, you will want to switch to short-blade fins and eventually to naked feet as you become more comfortable with doing various drills and exercises.

You will use each drill in the Green zone in the other zones. If you find you are having trouble with any specific drill, spend extra time to get it right. Often the real problem lies in having not mastered an earlier drill. Regardless of ability level, even the simplest drills described in this book will enhance the swimmer's neuromuscular knowledge.

Until you are familiar with each drill, you might want to photocopy the drill descriptions and put them in watertight sandwich bags so you can have them for quick reference at poolside while you practice.

Because most workout pools in the United States are 25 yards long, all workouts are for 25-yard pools. With minor adjustments, you may use them in 20-yard and 25-meter pools as well, and you can easily adapt most for 50-meter pools.

Reading the Workouts

There are some notation shortcuts used through the practice sections of this book. At first glance they may seem cryptic and confusing, but after you've read through the following examples you'll catch on quickly:

6 × 25 swim on :15R.   This means to swim 6 lengths (each length is 25 yards) of the pool, taking a full 15 seconds rest at each end of the pool.

6 × 25 swim on :15Rmax.   Same as previous example except Max (maximum) means you may opt to take less than 15 seconds rest if you desire. It is important to take enough rest so you recover and can execute the next length with good form.

6 × 25 on :15R—Alt 25 FB / 25 BB.   This means to go 6 lengths of the pool, taking 15 seconds rest after each length. Alternate one length of front balance drill and one length of back balance drill.

4 × 50 SGB on :15R—Alt 25Rt / 25Lft.   This means to do the SGB (side-glide balance) drill for 50 yards—2 lengths of the pool with no rest at the far end—then take 15 seconds rest, and repeat 3 times for a total of 4. On each 50, alternate the first length on your right side and the second length on your left side.

IHR.   Immediate heart rate—when you see this, take a heart rate as quickly as possible.

Good Versus Weak Side.   Many skills involve doing something on one side, then repeating the action on the other side (i.e., side-glide balance, breathing, etc.). You will usually find that you are better at performing the skill on one side than on the other. You'll be more relaxed, get into the proper position more quickly, be able to hold it longer and without as much effort, and so on. We call this your good side. The side on which you experience more problems is your weak side.

6 × :15 VK dry hands on :10R.   This notation asks for six 15-second periods of vertical kicking, while keeping both hands higher than the water surface. There are 10-second rests between each 15-second VK period.

Focus Points

When swimming rather than drilling, we don't want to turn off the brain and flail our arms and legs. So, for many swims, I have noted a specific sensation or mental image to focus on during the swim. These will include the following:

- **Downhill swimming:** Concentrate on holding the crown of your head in line with your spine as you maintain enough buoy pressure to keep your hips and legs at the surface. It should feel as though you are tilted slightly downward.

- **Long reach:** With each roll be aware that the arm entering the water continues to move forward to full extension as you complete the roll, as if reaching and stretching toward the far end of the pool.

- **Side skating:** Be aware that with each roll you get all the way onto your side, so your belly button points toward the side wall. Try to "skate" on that side for as long as possible before you begin the stroke with the extended arm.

- **Hand swapping:** Keep one arm extended in front of the body until the recovering or entering hand is ready to trade places. This is also called front quadrant swimming. See chapter 4, p. 42 for a description. The Glove is an exaggeration of this but is sometimes useful in getting the right feeling.

- **Marionette high elbow recovery:** See chapter 4, p. 47 for description.

- **Laser beam body-roll trigger:** See chapter 4, p. 47 for description.

- **Hip snap:** See chapter 4, p. 48 for description.

- **Vertical forearm stroke:** See chapter 4, p. 49 for description.

- **Stroke count:** Count the number of strokes it takes to swim each length of the pool. Count once for each hand as it enters the water. The last hand entry at the end of the pool counts as well, even though you touch the wall instead of taking another stroke.

As you go through the workout, move immediately from one activity to the next. Aim for no more than 15 to 20 seconds from completing one line of the workout until you begin the next line of the workout.

1

TOTAL TIME: 20-30 minutes

TARGET HEART RATE RANGE: 60-70% of max heart rate
RPE: 1-4
WARM-UP/COOL-DOWN: Do this entire practice at warm-up and cool-down intensity

WORKOUT

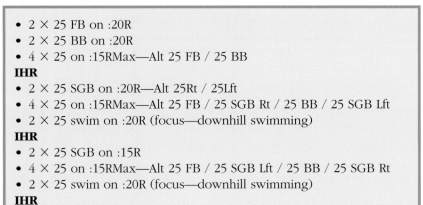

- 2 × 25 FB on :20R
- 2 × 25 BB on :20R
- 4 × 25 on :15RMax—Alt 25 FB / 25 BB

IHR

- 2 × 25 SGB on :20R—Alt 25Rt / 25Lft
- 4 × 25 on :15RMax—Alt 25 FB / 25 SGB Rt / 25 BB / 25 SGB Lft
- 2 × 25 swim on :20R (focus—downhill swimming)

IHR

- 2 × 25 SGB on :15R
- 4 × 25 on :15RMax—Alt 25 FB / 25 SGB Lft / 25 BB / 25 SGB Rt
- 2 × 25 swim on :20R (focus—downhill swimming)

IHR

TOTAL YARDAGE: 600 yards

COMMENTS

This is exclusively a static balance skills practice session. Do it all at an easy and comfortable pace. The focus is on executing each drill flawlessly and being as relaxed as possible. If you feel you need more rest, take it.

TOTAL TIME: 20-30 minutes

TARGET HEART RATE RANGE: 60-70% of max heart rate
RPE: 1-4
WARM-UP/COOL-DOWN: Do this entire practice at warm-up and cool-down intensity

WORKOUT

- 4 × 25 on :15RMax—Alt 25 FB / 25 BB
- 8 × 25 on :15RMax—Alt 25 FB / 25 SGB Rt / 25 BB / 25 SGB Lft
IHR
- 2 × 25 swim on :20R (focus—downhill swimming)
- 4 × 25 on :15RMax—Alt 25 FB / 25 SGB Lft / 25 BB / 25 SGB Rt
- 4 × :15 VK on :15R
IHR
- 4 × 25 on :15RMax—Alt 25 FB / 25 SGB Lft / 25 BB / 25 SGB Rt
- 4 × :15 VK on :10R
- 2 × 25 swim on :20R (focus—downhill swimming)
IHR

TOTAL YARDAGE: 750 yards (includes estimated yards for VK)

COMMENTS

This is almost exclusively a static balance skills practice session. Do it all at an easy and comfortable pace, except that the vertical kicking will likely be more intense. Focus on executing each drill flawlessly and being as relaxed as possible. Feel free to cut down the rest intervals on the drills you are more comfortable with, but if at any time you feel you need more rest, take it.

3

TOTAL TIME: 20-30 minutes

TARGET HEART RATE RANGE: 60-70% of max heart rate
RPE: 1-4
WARM-UP/COOL-DOWN: Do this entire practice at warm-up and cool-down intensity

WORKOUT

- 8 × 25 on :15RMax—Alt 25 FB / 25 SGB Rt / 25 BB / 25 SGB Lft
- 2 × 25 swim on :15R (focus—long reach)
- 2 × 25 BBR on :15R
IHR
- 1 × 25 SGB good side
- 2 × 25 SGBB on :15R good side
- 6 × :15 VK on :15R—Odd ones, hands on your chest; even ones, hands out of the water
- 2 × 25 BBR on :15R
- 1 × 25 SGB good side
IHR
- 2 × 25 SGB weak side
- 2 × 25 SGBB on :15R weak side
- 6 × :15 VK on :10R—Odd ones, hands on your chest; even ones, hands out of the water
- 2 × 25 swim on :20R (focus—downhill swimming)
IHR

TOTAL YARDAGE: 800 yards (includes estimated yards for VK)

COMMENTS

This practice includes both static and dynamic balance skills. As with the previous practices, do it all at an easy and comfortable pace, except the VK. The focus is still on flawless execution rather than speed. If you are using fins and feeling confident about some drills, you might want to try them with short-blade fins or with naked feet. Remember, the long-term goal is to be able to do all drills comfortably and relaxed without any fins.

STROKE INTEGRATION #1

TOTAL TIME: 20-30 minutes

TARGET HEART RATE RANGE: 60-70% of max heart rate
RPE: 1-4
WARM-UP

- 8 × 25 on :10R—Alt 25 BBR / 25 SGBB Rt / 25 BBR / 25 SGBB Lft
- 4 × 25 on :15RMax—Alt 25 SGBB / 25 swim (focus—side skating)
- IHR

WORKOUT

- 2 × 50 SGBB on :15R—Alt 25 good / 25 weak
- 2 × 25 SFS on :15RMax
- 2 × 25 SGBB on :10R—Alt 25 Rt / 25 Lft
- 2 × 25 SFS on :15RMax

IHR

- 4 × :20 VK on :10R—Odd ones, hands on your chest; even ones, hands out of the water

Cool-Down

- 6 × 25 on :15RMax—Alt 25 SGBB /25 SFS / 25 swim (focus—side skating)

IHR

TOTAL YARDAGE: 850 yards (includes estimated yards for VK)

COMMENTS

This practice introduces the first stroke integration drill, side-front-side (SFS), and still includes both static and dynamic balance skills. Note that some rest intervals have been shortened. As you get more skilled and relaxed at these drills, you should need less rest. However, the focus is still on flawless execution so, if you feel you need more rest to execute well, then take extra time at the walls.

5

TOTAL TIME: 20-30 minutes

TARGET HEART RATE RANGE: 60-70% of max heart rate

RPE: 1-4

WARM-UP

- 6 × 25 on :10R—Alt 25 SGBB Rt / 25 SGBB Lft / 25 SFS
- 4 × 25 on :10R—Alt 25 SFS / 25 swim (focus—side skating)
- IHR

WORKOUT

- 2 × 50 on :15RMax—Alt 25 SGBB / 25 SFS
- 4 × 25 on :10R—Alt 25 SFS / 25 SGF
- 2 × 50 on :15R—Alt 25 SGF / 25 SFS
- 2 × 25 swim on :10R (focus—side skating)

IHR

- 4 × :20 VK on :10R—Odd ones, hands on your chest; even ones, hands out of the water

Cool-Down

- 6 × 25 on :10R—Alt 25 SGBB /25 SFS / 25 swim (focus—side skating)

IHR

TOTAL YARDAGE: 900 yards (includes estimated yards for VK)

COMMENTS

This practice introduces another stroke integration drill, side-glide freestyle (SGF), and still includes dynamic balance skills. Take more rest than indicated if you are getting out of breath or if you need it to execute well. Have you been using short-blade fins or naked feet for some drills?

TOTAL TIME: 20-30 minutes

TARGET HEART RATE RANGE: 60-70% of max heart rate
RPE: 1-4
WARM-UP

- 4 × 25 on :10R—Alt 25 FB / 25 SGB Rt / 25 SGB Lft / 25 swim (focus—downhill swimming)
- 4 × 25 on :10R—Alt 25 BBR / 25 SGBB Rt / 25 SGBB Lft / 25 swim (focus—side skating)
- IHR

**W
O
R
K
O
U
T**

6

WORKOUT

- 2 × 25 on :15R 3&G
- 2 × 50 on :15RMax—Alt 25 SFS / 25 3&G
- 2 × 25 on :10R—Alt 25 SFS / 25 SGF
- 2 × 50 on :15R—Alt 25 SGF / 25 3&G (focus—vertical forearm stroke)

IHR

- 2 × 25 swim on :10R (focus—hand swapping)
- 4 × :20 VK on :10R—Odd ones, hands out of the water; even ones, hands on your head

IHR

Cool-Down

- 6 × 25 on :10R—Alt 25 SFS / 25 SGF / 25 swim (focus—hand swapping)

IHR

TOTAL YARDAGE: 850 yards (includes estimated yards for VK)

COMMENTS

This practice introduces the final stroke integration drill (3&G), along with a quick review of the earliest skills during the warm-up. Note that gradually you are increasing the amount of swimming. Reread the descriptions of the focus points indicated for each swim. Note the change in hand and arm positions on the VK set.

7 WORKOUT

TOTAL TIME: 20-30 minutes

TARGET HEART RATE RANGE: 60-70% of max heart rate

RPE: 1-4

WARM-UP

- 4 × 25 on :10R—Alt 25 SGB Rt / 25 SGB Lft / 25 SFS / 25 swim (focus—side skating)
- 4 × 25 on :10R—Alt 25 SGBB Rt / 25 SGBB Lft / 25 SGF / 25 swim (focus—hand swapping)
- IHR

WORKOUT

- 2 × 50 on :15RMax—Alt 25 SFS / 25 3&G (focus—vertical forearm stroke)
- 2 × 25 SGF on :10R
- 2 × 75 on :30RMax—Alt 25 SFS / 25 3&G / 25 swim (focus—hand swapping)

IHR

- 1 × 25 FB
- 1 × 25 BB
- 4 × :30 VK on :15R—Odd ones, hands out of the water; even ones, hands on your head

IHR

Cool-Down

- 3 × 50 on :10R—Alt 25 BB / 25 SGBB

IHR

TOTAL YARDAGE: 900 yards (includes estimated yards for VK)

COMMENTS

This practice includes at least one length of each skill drill. Note that gradually we are stringing together longer series of drill and swim lengths without rest. The VK part of this workout is the most demanding yet.

ADDING SOME SPEED

TOTAL TIME: 20-30 minutes

TARGET HEART RATE RANGE: 60-70% of max heart rate
RPE: 1-4
WARM-UP

- 4 × 25 on :10R—Alt 25 SFS / 25 SGB weak / 25 SFS / 25 swim (focus—side skating)
- 2 × 50 on :10R—Alt 25 SGBB weak / 25 swim (focus—hip snap)
- IHR

WORKOUT

- 1 × 100—Alt 25 FB / 25 SGBB weak / 25 3&G / 25 swim (focus—hip snap)
- 1 × 75 SGB—Alt 25 weak / 25 good / 25 weak
- 1 × 75—Alt 25 SFS / 25 3&G / 25 swim (focus—hand swapping)
- 1 × 50 SGB—Alt 25 weak / 25 good

IHR

- 1 × 25 swim fast (focus—downhill swimming)
- 1 × 25 SGBB weak
- 1 × 25 swim fast (focus—hip snap)
- 1 × 25 SGB weak
- 4 × :15 VK on :15R—Hands on your head

IHR
Cool-Down

- 3 × 50 on :10R—Alt 25 SGBB weak / 25 SGBB good

IHR

TOTAL YARDAGE: 900 yards (includes estimated yards for VK)

COMMENTS

This is the first practice in which you swim fast on a couple lengths. Don't be alarmed if all your new technique improvements seem to fall apart the first few times you swim fast—this is normal. Take extra rest after these if you need to. Also, note the emphasis on side-glide drills on your weak side? Try to pinpoint what you are doing differently on your weak side that prevents it from feeling like your good side. This usually is a problem with head position, buoy pressure, or both.

TOTAL TIME: 20-30 minutes

TARGET HEART RATE RANGE: 60-70% of max heart rate
RPE: 1-4
WARM-UP
- 4 × 25 on :10R—Alt 25 SFS / 25 SGB weak / 25 SFS / 25 swim (focus—side skating)
- 2 × 50 on :10R—Alt 25 SGBB weak / 25 swim (focus—hip snap)
- IHR

WORKOUT

- 1 × 100—Alt 25 FB / 25 SGBB weak / 25 5&G / 25 swim (focus—hand swapping)
- 2 × 75 on :15RMax—Alt 25 5&G / 25 SFS / 25 5&G (focus—vertical forearm stroke)
- 2 × 50 on :10RMax—Alt 25 SFS / 25 swim (focus—marionette high elbow recovery)

IHR
- 1 × 25 SGF
- 1 × 25 swim fast (focus—long reach)
- 1 × 25 SGBB weak
- 1 × 25 swim fast (focus—side skating)
- 1 × 25 SGBB good
- 3 × 25 swim (focus—laser beam body-roll trigger) on :15RMax

IHR
Cool-Down
- 3 × 50 on :10R—Alt 25 SGB weak / 25 5&G

IHR

TOTAL YARDAGE: 900 yards

Be sure to reread the description for each focus point for the swims in this practice—then apply it. Turning your brain off (or, conversely, trying to focus on 15 things at once) decreases your ability to perform well and your neuromuscular learning potential.

TOTAL TIME: 20-30 minutes

TARGET HEART RATE RANGE: 60-70% of max heart rate
RPE: 1-4
WARM-UP

- 4 × 50 on :10R—Alt 25 SGBB weak / 25 5&G
- 2 × 50 on :10R—Alt 25 SGBB good / 25 swim (focus—stroke count)
- IHR

WORKOUT

- 1 × 100—Alt 25 SGBB good / 25 3&G / 25 5&G / 25 swim (focus—stroke count)
- 2 × 75 on :10RMax—Alt 25 SGF / 25 5&G / 25 swim (focus—stroke count)
- 2 × 50 on :10RMax—Alt 25 SGF / 25 swim (focus—stroke count)
- 1 × 25 swim fast (focus—hand swapping and stroke count)
- 1 × 25 SGBB weak

IHR
- 1 × 25 swim fast (focus—side skating and stroke count)
- 1 × 25 3&G
- 4 × 25 swim on :15RMax—Each one faster than the previous one (focus—1 long reach, 2 hand swapping, 3 downhill swimming, 4 hip snap, and stroke count on all 4)

IHR
Cool-Down
- 3 × 50 on :10R—Alt 25 SGB weak / 25 5&G

IHR

TOTAL YARDAGE: 1,000 yards

COMMENTS

Move from one line of the workout to the next as quickly as possible. Note the emphasis on stroke counting in this practice. Stroke count is our most useful and immediate feedback tool for swimming efficiency. We're always looking to lower stroke counts at all speeds. As speed increases we want to overcome the tendency to increase the number of strokes we take for each length.

Before You Move to the Blue Zone

After you have completed all the practices in the Green zone once, repeat the T-15 swim from chapter 3. The idea is to go farther in the allotted 15-minute period. Do the T-15 without fins so you'll be comparing apples to apples.

If you were unable to complete the initial T-15 swim without stopping, then you may have a significant improvement by simply taking shorter rests. You will also want to spend much of your swimming time emphasizing the fundamentals you have been learning. Use the focus points throughout the swim to keep your gray matter properly engaged—downhill swimming, long reach, side skating, hand swapping, marionette high elbow recovery, laser beam body-roll trigger, hip snap, and stroke count.

After you complete the T-15, record your results with your original results. Each time you go through a complete set of practices in a color, do another T-15 swim. If you decide to go back through the Green practices again, repeat the T-15 and record the results before going on to the Blue zone.

Blue Zone

Assuming you have worked through the complete set of Green zone practices a couple times and can complete them easily and within your target heart rate range, it is probably time to move to the Blue zone practices. By now you should feel confident about the skill drills and focus points in the Green zone. If not, you may want to review and practice in the areas you are concerned about.

Practices in the Blue zone, like those in the Green zone, consist primarily of body balance and swimming skill drills with a small amount of full-stroke swimming. The duration of these practices will be longer (30-40 minutes rather than 20-30 minutes for the Green zone). These practices are similar to the Green zone practices except there are more repetitions of the drills and some different focus points.

Although I still encourage training fins for any drills you have not yet become comfortable with, our long-term goal is to move from long-blade fins to short-blade fins and, finally, to naked feet in all drills. As you work through these practices, always look for opportunities to rely less on fins, especially when swimming rather than drilling.

Reading the Workouts

This section introduces a few new notation shortcuts:

4 × 25 swim 1@NS/L, 2@–1S/L, 1@–2S/L.   S/L is strokes per length. There will be more stroke-counting activity in the Blue zone, so you will need to be aware of and control how many strokes per length you are taking. By 1@NS/L, I mean to swim one 25 at normal S/L—the number of strokes per length you are taking *right now* when you are not trying to do anything special. By 2@–1S/L, I mean to swim the next two 25s at one fewer strokes than normal count (same idea for –2S/L, –3S/L, etc.). In this example, if you swim the first 25 with a stroke count of 18, then the next two lengths should be at 17 strokes, and the fourth at 16.

4 ×25 swim—Descend 1-4 (or desc 1-4).   The Blue zone introduces a few series of swims in which you vary your speed. Descend 1-4 means that in a set of 4 swims, do the first one at an easy pace, the second one a bit faster, the third even faster, and the fourth one faster still.

6 ×25 swim—Desc 1-3 Rpt.   Descend 1-3 repeatedly—descend swims 1 through 3, then on number 4 go back to a slower pace and begin descending again.

New Focus Point

Here is one more mental image to use as a focus point while swimming or drilling:

- **Skewer:** Stand up straight, look straight ahead, and imagine a skewer piercing down through the crown of your head and along the length of your spine. When you swim, imagine this skewer always in place and your job is to never do anything that would bend the skewer. When you rotate your body from one side-glide position to the other side-glide position, that skewer should be the axis of rotation. When you turn your head to breathe, that skewer is the axis of rotation. If you lift your head, even a bit, you'll bend the skewer. Anytime you bend the skewer, you get out of balance.

Now enter the Blue zone.

STATIC BALANCE

TOTAL TIME: 30-40 minutes

TARGET HEART RATE RANGE: 60-70% of max heart rate
RPE: 1-4
WARM-UP/COOL-DOWN: Do this entire practice at warm-up and cool-down intensity

WORKOUT

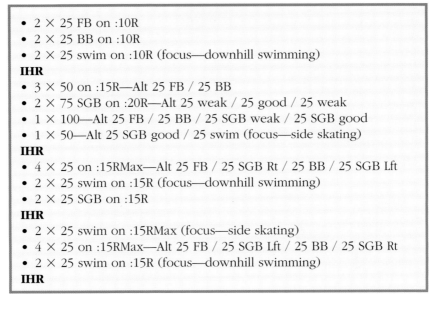

- 2 × 25 FB on :10R
- 2 × 25 BB on :10R
- 2 × 25 swim on :10R (focus—downhill swimming)

IHR

- 3 × 50 on :15R—Alt 25 FB / 25 BB
- 2 × 75 SGB on :20R—Alt 25 weak / 25 good / 25 weak
- 1 × 100—Alt 25 FB / 25 BB / 25 SGB weak / 25 SGB good
- 1 × 50—Alt 25 SGB good / 25 swim (focus—side skating)

IHR

- 4 × 25 on :15RMax—Alt 25 FB / 25 SGB Rt / 25 BB / 25 SGB Lft
- 2 × 25 swim on :15R (focus—downhill swimming)
- 2 × 25 SGB on :15R

IHR

- 2 × 25 swim on :15RMax (focus—side skating)
- 4 × 25 on :15RMax—Alt 25 FB / 25 SGB Lft / 25 BB / 25 SGB Rt
- 2 × 25 swim on :15R (focus—downhill swimming)

IHR

TOTAL YARDAGE: 1,000 yards

COMMENTS

Just like the first practice in the Green zone, this is exclusively a static balance skills practice session. The focus is on executing each drill flawlessly, as comfortably and relaxed as possible. If you feel you need more rest, take it.

2

TOTAL TIME: 30-40 minutes

TARGET HEART RATE RANGE: 60-70% of max heart rate

RPE: 1-4

WARM-UP/COOL-DOWN: Do this entire practice at warm-up and cool-down intensity

WORKOUT

- 4 × 25 on :15RMax—Alt 25 FB / 25 BB
- 8 × 25 on :15RMax—Alt 25 FB / 25 SGB Rt / 25 BB / 25 SGB Lft
- 4 × 25 on :15R—Alt 25 SGB good / 25 swim (focus—downhill swimming)

IHR

- 4 × 25 on :15RMax—Alt 25 FB / 25 SGB Lft / 25 BB / 25 SGB Rt
- 4 × :15 VK on :10R—Hands on your chest
- 6 × 25 on :15RMax—Alt 25 FB / 25 SGB weak / 25 swim (focus—side skating)

IHR

- 4 × :15 VK on :10R—Hands out of water
- 4 × 25 swim on :15RMax (focus—25 downhill swimming / 25 side skating)
- 6 × :15 VK on :10R—Hands out of water
- 2 × 50 on :15RMax—Alt 25 SGB weak / 25 swim (focus—stroke count)

IHR

TOTAL YARDAGE: 1,100 yards (includes estimated yards for VK)

COMMENTS

Again, this is mainly a static balance skills practice session. Keep it easy (except the VK might be more intense), cutting down the rest intervals on the drills you are comfortable on. Are you making enough progress on these simplest drills to cut down on fin use?

BALANCE

TOTAL TIME: 30-40 minutes

TARGET HEART RATE RANGE: 60-70% of max heart rate
RPE: 1-4
WARM-UP

- 8 × 25 on :15RMax—Alt 25 FB / 25 SGB Rt / 25 BB / 25 SGB Lft
- 2 × 25 swim on :15R (focus—long reach)
- IHR

WORKOUT

- 4 × 25 swim on :20RMax—Descend 1-3 (focus—stroke count; don't let the S/L go up)
- 2 × 25 BBR on :15R
- 3 × 25 SGB on :10R—Alt 25 weak / 25 good / 25 weak
- 3 × 25 SGBB on :15R—Alt 25 weak / 25 good / 25 weak

IHR

- 6 × :15 VK on :15R—Odd ones, hands on your chest; even ones, hands out of the water

IHR

- 2 × 25 BBR on :15R
- 6 × 25 SGBB on :15R—Alt 25 weak / 25 good / 25 swim (focus—skewer)
- 2 × 25 SGB on :15R weak

IHR

- 6 × :15 VK on :10R—Odd ones, hands on your chest; even ones, hands out of the water

IHR
Cool-Down

- 2 × 25 swim on :15R (focus—downhill swimming)
- 2 × 25 BBR on :10R

IHR

TOTAL YARDAGE: 1,200 yards (includes estimated yards for VK)

COMMENTS

Note that often you do a drill to isolate a skill, then follow it with a swim in which some aspect of that skill is the focal point. This accelerates the neuromuscular learning process. Have you tried any of the VK with short-blade fins or no fins?

4

W
O
R
K
O
U
T

TOTAL TIME: 30-40 minutes

TARGET HEART RATE RANGE: 60-70% of max heart rate
RPE: 1-4
WARM-UP

- 8 × 25 on :10R—Alt 25 BBR / 25 SGBB Rt / 25 BBR / 25 SGBB Lft
- 4 × 25 on :15RMax—Alt 25 SGBB / 25 swim (focus—side skating and stroke count)
- IHR

WORKOUT

- 4 × 75 SGBB on :20R—Alt 25 good / 25 weak / swim (focus—skewer)
- 4 × 25 SFS on :15RMax
- 2 × 25 SGBB on :10R—Alt 25 Rt / 25 Lft
- 2 × 25 SFS on :15RMax (focus—vertical forearm stroke)
- 2 × 25 swim on :15R (focus—side skating and stroke count)

IHR

- 6 × :20 VK on :15R—Odd ones, hands on your chest; even ones, hands out of the water

Cool-Down

- 6 × 25 on :15RMax—Alt 25 SGBB /25 SFS / 25 swim (focus—side skating)

IHR

TOTAL YARDAGE: 1,200 yards (includes estimated yards for VK)

COMMENTS

As you get more skilled and relaxed at these drills, you should need less rest. See how little rest you can get away with on those that ask for RMax rest. However, the focus is still on flawless execution, so if you feel you need more rest to execute well, then take extra time. Always take some aspect of a drill you have mastered and duplicate it in your full-stroke swimming.

STROKE INTEGRATION #2

TOTAL TIME: 30-40 minutes

TARGET HEART RATE RANGE: 60-70% of max heart rate
RPE: 1-4
WARM-UP

- 6 × 25 on :10R—Alt 25 SGBB Rt / 25 SGBB Lft / 25 swim (focus—skewer)
- 6 × 25 on :10R—Alt 25 SFS / 25 swim (focus—side skating)
- IHR

WORKOUT

- 6 × 50 on :15RMax—Alt 50 SGBB / 50 SFS / 50 5&G
- 4 × 25 on :10R—Alt 25 SGF / 25 swim (focus—hand swapping)
- 2 × 50 on :15R—Alt 25 SGF / 25 SFS (focus—vertical forearm stroke)
- 2 × 25 swim on :10R (focus—side skating and stroke count) 1@NS/L, 1@–2S/L

IHR
- 4 × :20 VK on :10R—Odd ones, hands on your chest; even ones, hands out of the water

IHR
Cool-Down
- 6 × 25 on :10R—Alt 25 SGBB /25 SFS / 25 swim (focus—side skating)

IHR

TOTAL YARDAGE: 1,300 yards (includes estimated yards for VK)

COMMENTS

Take more rest than indicated if you are getting out of breath or if you feel you need it to execute well. On which drills have you been using short-blade fins or naked feet? I hope all your static balance drills (FB, BB, SGB) and perhaps your dynamic balance drills (BBR, SGBB) are at this point.

6 WORKOUT

TOTAL TIME: 30-40 minutes

TARGET HEART RATE RANGE: 60-70% of max heart rate
RPE: 1-4
WARM-UP
- 4 × 25 on :10R—Alt 25 FB / 25 SGB Rt / 25 SGB Lft / 25 swim (focus—downhill swimming)
- 4 × 25 on :10R—Alt 25 BBR / 25 SGBB Rt / 25 SGBB Lft / 25 swim (focus—side skating)
- 4 × 25 on :10R—Alt 25 SFS / 25 3&G / 25 5&G / 25 swim (focus—hand swapping)
- IHR

WORKOUT

- 2 × 25 swim on :10R (focus—marionette high elbow recovery and laser beam body-roll trigger)
- 2 × 50 on :15RMax—Alt 25 SFS / 25 3&G
- 2 × 25 on :10RMax—Alt 25 SFS / 25 SGF (focus—vertical forearm stroke)
- 4 × 75 on :15R—Alt 25 SGF / 25 3&G / 25 swim (focus—side skating)
IHR
- 2 × 25 swim on :10R (focus—hand swapping)
- 4 × :20 VK on :10R—Odd ones, hands out of the water; even ones, hands on your head
IHR
Cool-Down
- 6 × 25 on :10R—Alt 25 SFS / 25 SGF / 25 swim (focus—hand swapping and stroke count)
IHR

TOTAL YARDAGE: 1,200 yards (includes estimated yards for VK)

COMMENTS

Be sure to reread the descriptions of the focus points for each swim. Note the change in hand and arm positions on the VK set.

DRILL REVIEW

TOTAL TIME: 30-40 minutes

TARGET HEART RATE RANGE: 60-70% of max heart rate
RPE: 1-4
WARM-UP

- 4 × 25 on :10R—Alt 25 SGB Rt / 25 SGB Lft / 25 SFS / 25 swim (focus—side skating)
- 4 × 50 on :15R—Alt 25 SGF / 25 swim (focus—hand swapping)
- IHR

WORKOUT

- 2 × 50 on :15RMax—Alt 25 SFS / 25 3&G
- 2 × 25 SGF on :10R (focus—vertical forearm stroke)
- 2 × 75 on :30RMax—Alt 25 SFS / 25 3&G / 25 swim (focus—hand swapping)

IHR

- 1 × 25 FB
- 2 × 25 swim on :5R (focus—downhill swimming) 1@NS/L, 1@–2S/L
- 1 × 25 SGF (focus—skewer)
- 2 × 25 swim on :5R (focus—side skating) 1@NS/L, 1@–2S/L
- 4 × :30 VK on :10R—Odd ones, hands out of the water; even ones, hands on your head

IHR
Cool-Down

- 4 × 75 on :15R—Alt 25 BB / 25 SGBB / 25 swim (focus—stroke count)

IHR

TOTAL YARDAGE: 1,300 yards (includes estimated yards for VK)

COMMENTS

This practice includes at least one length of each skill drill. Regardless of conditioning or ability level, every time you revisit a drill that your brain thinks you already know well, your neuromuscular system learns new skills or refines old ones. The VK part of this workout is the most demanding yet.

8

TOTAL TIME: 30-40 minutes

TARGET HEART RATE RANGE: 60-70% of max heart rate

RPE: 1-4

WARM-UP

- 4 × 25 on :10R—Alt 25 SFS / 25 SGB weak / 25 SFS / 25 swim (focus—side skating)
- 2 × 50 on :10R—Alt 25 SGBB weak / 25 swim (focus—hip snap)
- 1 × 100—Alt 50 swim (focus—stroke count NS/L) / 25 SGB weak / 25 swim (focus—stroke count –2S/L)
- IHR

WORKOUT

- 1 × 100—Alt 25 FB / 25 SGBB weak / 25 3&G / 25 swim (focus—hip snap)
- 2 × 75 SGB on :10RMax—Alt 25 weak / 25 good / 25 weak
- 2 × 75 on :15RMax—Alt 25 SFS / 25 3&G / 25 swim (focus—hand swapping)
- 3 × 50 SGB on :10RMax—Alt 25 weak / 25 good

IHR

- 1 × 25 swim fast (focus—downhill swimming)
- 1 × 25 SGBB weak
- 1 × 25 swim fast (focus—hip snap)
- 1 × 25 SGB weak
- 4 × :15 VK on :15R— Hands on your head

IHR

Cool-Down

- 3 × 50 on :10R—Alt 25 SGBB weak / 25 swim (focus—skewer)

IHR

TOTAL YARDAGE: 1,300 yards (includes estimated yards for VK)

COMMENTS

It has been a while since you've swum fast on a couple lengths. You should be noticing a few skills showing up in your faster swimming. Take extra rest after these if you need to. Pinpoint what you are doing differently on your weak side drills that prevents them from feeling like your good side. This usually is a problem with head position, buoy pressure, or both.

FOCUSED SWIMMING

TOTAL TIME: 30-40 minutes

TARGET HEART RATE RANGE: 60-70% of max heart rate
RPE: 1-4
WARM-UP

- 4 × 25 on :10R—Alt 25 SFS / 25 SGB weak / 25 SFS / 25 swim (focus—side skating)
- 4 × 50 on :10R—Alt 25 SGBB weak / 25 swim (focus—hip snap)
- IHR

WORKOUT

- 3 × 100 on :20R—Alt 25 FB / 25 SGBB weak / 25 5&G / 25 swim (focus—hand swapping and stroke count)
- 3 × 75 on :15RMax—Alt 25 5&G / 25 SFS / 25 5&G
- 3 × 50 on :10RMax—Alt 25 SFS / 25 swim (focus—marionette high elbow recovery)

IHR
- 1 × 25 SGF
- 1 × 25 swim fast (focus—long reach) NS/L
- 1 × 25 SGBB weak
- 1 × 25 swim fast (focus—side skating) –1S/L

IHR
- 1 × 25 SGBB good
- 1 × 25 swim fast (focus—hand swapping)
- 1 × 25 SGF (focus—vertical forearm stroke)
- 4 × 25 swim (focus—laser beam body-roll trigger and stroke count) on :15RMax

IHR
Cool-Down
- 3 × 50 on :10R—Alt 25 SGB weak / 25 5&G

IHR

TOTAL YARDAGE: 1,400 yards

COMMENTS

Do you know what each focus point means? If you don't know one well enough to teach it to someone else, then go back and study the description. This practice has more full-stroke swimming in it than any so far. Are your stroke counts lower than when you started these practices?

COUNT AWARENESS

10

WORKOUT

TOTAL TIME: 30-40 minutes

TARGET HEART RATE RANGE: 60-70% of max heart rate

RPE: 1-4

WARM-UP

- 4 × 50 on :10R—Alt 25 SGBB weak / 25 5&G
- 2 × 50 on :10R—Alt 25 SGBB good / 25 swim (focus—stroke count)
- IHR

WORKOUT

- 4 × :15 VK on :10RMax
- 1 × 100—Alt 25 SGBB good / 25 3&G / 25 5&G / 25 swim (focus—stroke count)
- 2 × 75 on :10RMax—Alt 25 SGF / 25 5&G / 25 swim (focus—stroke count)
- 2 × 50 on :10RMax—Alt 25 SGF / 25 swim (focus—stroke count)
- 2 × 25 swim fast on :30R (focus—hip snap and stroke count)
- 4 × 25 on :10RMax—Alt 25 SGBB weak / 25 SGBB good

IHR

- 4 × 25 swim on :15RMax (focus—side skating and stroke count) 1@NS/L, 2@–1S/L, 1@–2S/L
- 2 × 25 3&G on :5R
- 4 × 50 swim on :30RMax—Descend 1-4 (focus—1 long reach, 2 hand swapping, 3 downhill swimming, 4 hip snap, and stroke count on all 4)

IHR

Cool-Down

- 3 × 50 on :10R—Alt 25 SGB weak / 25 5&G

IHR

TOTAL YARDAGE: 1,400 yards

COMMENTS

Move from one line of the workout to the next as quickly as possible. Note the emphasis on stroke counting in this practice. Lowering stroke counts at all speeds should be a continuous process. This practice has the longest string of uninterrupted swimming (4 × 50 descending) so far. You'll have to start this series at a slower pace than you might think to descend the times.

8

Purple Zone

In the Blue zone you continued a focus on learning and refining skill drills in a workout format. The amount of swimming was restricted to no more than 30 percent of the yardage of any practice. If you have gone through the Blue zone a couple times and can stay within your target heart rate range most of the time (except when a fast swim or vertical kicking was indicated), it is time to enter the Purple zone.

Practices in the Purple zone will involve more full-stroke swimming but will still include from 30-percent to 50-percent skill drills. The duration of these practices will remain in the 30- to 40-minute range. However, the intensity will be increasing, either by reducing rest or increasing speed, so the total yardage you cover in these practices will be greater than in the Blue zone.

Although I encourage training fins for drills you have not yet become comfortable with, you should have at least moved to short-blade fins for these. Beginning now, the practice notation will include information about when to use fins. Except for using short-blade fins on drills you still need them for, do not use fins unless the practice notation calls for them.

Reading the Workouts

This section introduces a few new notation shortcuts:

Fins

The following practice sets involve the use of fins.

4 × 25 swim Fins

4 × 25 swim SBFins

4 × 25 swim FinsOpt

When the word fins appears, use full-blade fins. SBFins refers to short-blade fins. FinsOpt means that you may wear fins or not as you choose.

DChoice

DChoice means drill choice. Where this appears, you may substitute any skill drill I have presented. Here's what you'll see:

4 × 25 on :10R DChoice

4 × 25 on :10R SBDChoice

4 × 25 on :10R DBDChoice

4 × 25 on :10R SIDChoice

4 × 25 on :10R DChoiceMix

SBDChoice means your choice of the static balance drills (FB, BB, SGB). DBDChoice refers to our dynamic balance drills (SGBB, BBR). SIDChoice is choice of stroke integration drills (SFS, SGF, 3&G, 5&G). DChoiceMix means you may choose and mix more than one drill, perhaps going one length of FB, one length of SGB, and two lengths of 3&G.

Some More Workout Sets

Don't think you're getting off that easily. Here are a few more workout set notations that you'll see in the Purple Zone.

8-minute set of 50s swim (focus—stroke count) on IHR (keep HR in target range). Swim a 50, focusing on stroke count. Take an immediate heart rate. As soon as you know the IHR, swim another 50, take another IHR, and repeat this pattern until 8 minutes is up. If you have time before the 8 minutes is up to start another 50, do the whole 50. On this set, the final instruction asks you to swim at a pace that keeps your IHR continuously in the target heart rate range for this practice.

4 × 50 swim fast on 2:00 (or on 1:00RMin). Swim four 50s fast on a 2-minute interval (start a new 50 every 2 minutes). In parenthesis there is an alternative for slower swimmers—1:00RMin means you should get at least 1 minute rest. If a 2-minute interval doesn't allow at least 1 minute rest, then go on a longer interval that does allow a full minute or more rest. With long rests like this we mean active rest. You should keep moving and improve recovery—either easy swimming, treading water, or other low-intensity water exercises.

4 × 50 SGolf on 2:00.   Swim four 50s on a 2-minute interval. For each 50, count total strokes you take in the swim, note your elapsed swim time on the clock, and use part of the rest period to compute your swimming golf (SGolf) score for the swim. The idea in any SGolf set is to keep lowering your score. (See chapter 3, p. 27 for a detailed description of swimming golf.)

New Focus Point

Swimming involves a never-ending learning and refinement process. With that in mind, I offer another concept to cogitate from time to time as you stare at the black line:

- **Hands and hips connection:** You might recall from chapter 4 (Swimming on Your Sides, p. 39) that the swimming engine for truly effective swimming is in the hips, not the arms. Like the baseball pitcher, we want to use our arms primarily to transmit the large forces generated by hip roll to the water. An effective thought picture to develop is keeping a connection of the hand to the hip on the same side of the body. In a literal sense, the hip and hand are connected indirectly via bones, muscles, and connective tissue. What we want to do is exploit that connection.

If you are executing front quadrant swimming, you will keep one arm extended underwater in front of you until the recovering arm nearly catches up to it. At the moment your recovering arm passes your head on its way to entry, the hips should begin to roll. An instant *after* that, the extended arm begins to take the stroke as the body rolls with the hips. Timed in this manner, you should feel as though your extended arm is being tugged back slightly by the hip *before* you begin the arm stroke. Then your shoulder and arm muscles should put only as much pressure on your hand as is necessary to complete the stroke at the same instant that the hip and body roll reaches completion. You should be able to feel a connection of the hip to the hand throughout the stroke. If you start stroking too early, you will not feel this connection. Likewise, if you work too hard with the arm and shoulder, putting too much pressure on the hand, the stroke will get ahead of the roll and you will not feel the connection (an analogous scenario would be a baseball pitcher throwing the ball, starting with her arm motion first, then later turning her hips).

We also want to maintain a feeling of connection between the entering arm and its hip. As the recovering arm passes the head and begins the entry phase, you should feel as though the hand slices forward to full extension as a result of the body roll, rather than just stabbing the hand forward from the shoulder. The extension of the arm forward starts as the body begins to roll and ends as the body roll reaches completion. On to the Purple zone.

1

TOTAL TIME: 30-40 minutes

TARGET HEART RATE RANGE: 70-85% of max heart rate

RPE: 4-7

WARM-UP

- 4 × 50 on :10R—Alt 25 DChoice / 25 swim SBFinsOpt
- 4 × 25 3&G on :10RMax
- IHR

WORKOUT

- 4 × 25 swim on :10R (focus—downhill swimming) descend 1-4
- 1 × 150 SBFinsOpt—Alt 50 3&G / 50 5&G / 50 swim (focus—side skating)
- 4 × 50 on :15R—Alt 25 3&G / 25 swim (focus—stroke count, odd ones @NS/L, evens @–2S/L)
- 3 × 100 on :20RMax—Alt 25 SGBB weak / swim 25 (focus—skewer) / 25 SGBB good / swim 25 (focus—skewer)

IHR

Cool-Down

- 2 × 25 swim on :15RMax (focus—side skating) 1@NS/L, 1@–2S/L
- 4 × 25 on :15RMax FinsOpt—Alt 25 FB / 25 SGB Lft / 25 BB / 25 SGB Rt
- 2 × 25 swim on :15R (focus—downhill swimming) both @–1S/L

IHR

TOTAL YARDAGE: 1,250 yards

COMMENTS

This practice has more full-stroke swimming in it than any of the Green or Blue practices. Emphasize doing each swim well rather than fast. As some swim and drill combinations get longer, it is important to turn quickly at the walls and get a good, long, streamlined push-off.

VERTICAL KICKING

TOTAL TIME: 30-40 minutes

TARGET HEART RATE RANGE: 70-85% of max heart rate
RPE: 4-7
WARM-UP

- 4 × 25 on :10RMax FinsOpt—Alt 25 FB / 25 swim (focus—downhill swimming)
- 4 × 25 on :10RMax SBFins—Alt 25 SGB Rt / 25 SGBB Rt / 25 SGB Lft / 25 SGBB Lft
- 4 × 25 on :10R—Alt 25 SGB good / 25 swim (focus—downhill swimming)
- IHR

WORKOUT

- 4 × 25 on :15RMax—Alt 25 FB / 25 SGB good / 25 BB / 25 swim (focus—stroke count)

IHR
- 4 × :15 VK on :10R—Hands on your chest

IHR
- 6 × 75 on :10RMax SBFinsOpt—Alt 25 FB / 25 SGB weak / 25 swim (focus—side skating)

IHR
- 6 × :15 VK SBFins on :10R—Dry hands

IHR
- 4 × 25 swim on :15RMax (focus—25 downhill swimming / 25 side skating)

IHR
- 6 × :15 VK Fins on :10R—Dry elbows and hands

IHR
Cool-Down
- 2 × 100 on :15RMax—Alt 25 SGBB weak / 25 swim (focus—stroke count)

TOTAL YARDAGE: 1,300 yards (includes estimated yards for VK)

COMMENTS

Play with the size and speed of your kick to see how little you can let your HR rise on those VK sets. As you progress through the Purple practices, go from one set or activity to the next as quickly as possible. Ideally, you should have short enough breaks between each activity that your heart rate never goes below the 120 to 130 range during the entire practice. Taking too much rest decreases the aerobic benefit of the workout.

STROKE COUNTING

TOTAL TIME: 30-40 minutes

TARGET HEART RATE RANGE: 70-85% of max heart rate

RPE: 4-7

WARM-UP

- 8 × 25 on :15RMax FinsOpt—Alt 25 FB / 25 SGB Rt / 25 BB / 25 SGB Lft
- 2 × 75 swim on :20R (focus—25 long reach / 25 marionette high elbow recovery / 25 laser beam body-roll trigger)
- IHR

WORKOUT

- 10 × 25 on :15RMax—Alt 25 3&G / 25 swim (focus—stroke count; don't let the S/L go up as the set progresses)

IHR

- 5 × 50 on :15RMax—Alt 25 5&G / 25 swim (focus—stroke count; don't let the S/L go up as the set progresses)

IHR

- 8 × :15 VK SBFins on :15R—Odd ones, hands on your chest; even ones, dry hands and elbows

IHR

- 1 × 100 swim (focus—stroke count; don't let it go up from length to length)

IHR

Cool-Down

- 6 × 25 swim on :10R (focus—downhill swimming) 2@NS/L, 2@–2S/L, 2@–3S/L
- 4 × 25 DChoice SBFins on :10R

IHR

TOTAL YARDAGE: 1,350 yards (includes estimated yards for VK)

COMMENTS

Longest sets yet appear in this practice. You could do the VK activity that calls for dry elbows and hands in full streamline stretch position (see chapter 5, p. 59 for description).

TOTAL TIME: 30-40 minutes

TARGET HEART RATE RANGE: 70-85% of max heart rate
RPE: 4-7
WARM-UP

- 4 × 25 on :10R Fins—Alt 25 BBR / 25 SGBB Rt / 25 BBR / 25 SGBB Lft
- 4 × 25 on :10R SBFins—Alt 25 BBR / 25 SGBB Rt / 25 BBR / 25 SGBB Lft
- 4 × 25 on :10R—Alt 25 BBR / 25 SGBB Rt / 25 BBR / 25 SGBB Lft
- 1 × 100—Alt 25 SGBB / 25 swim (focus—side skating and stroke count)
- IHR

WORKOUT

- 8-minute set of 50s swim (focus—stroke count) on IHR (keep HR in target range)
- 1 × 50 SFS (focus—hand/hip connection)
- 1 × 50 SGBB—Alt 25 Rt / 25 Lft

IHR

- 1 × 50 SFS (focus—vertical forearm stroke)
- 1 × 50 swim (focus—side skating and stroke count)

IHR

- 6 × :20 VK on :15R—Odd ones, hands on your chest; even ones, dry hands

IHR

Cool-Down

- 4 × 75 on :15RMax SBFins—Alt 25 SGBB /25 SFS / 25 swim (focus—hand/hip connection)

IHR

TOTAL YARDAGE: approximately 1,400 yards (includes estimated yards for VK)

COMMENTS

Note that there are fewer 25s and more long drills and swims. As you get more skilled and relaxed at these drills, you should need less rest. Always take some aspect of a drill you have mastered and duplicate it in your full-stroke swimming. Did you try that VK with smaller or no fins?

W
O
R
K
O
U
T

5

TOTAL TIME: 30-40 minutes

TARGET HEART RATE RANGE: 70-85% of max heart rate

RPE: 4-7

WARM-UP

- 4 × 75 on :15R SBFins—Alt 25 SGBB Rt / 25 SGBB Lft / 25 swim (focus—skewer)
- IHR

WORKOUT

- 6 × 50 on :15RMax—Alt 50 SFS / 50 SGF / 50 3&G (focus—hand/hip connection)

IHR

- 6 × 50 on :15R Fins—Alt 25 3&G / 25 swim fast (focus—side skating)

IHR

- 8 × :20 VK on :10R—Odd ones, dry hands; even ones, dry hands and elbows

IHR

Cool-Down

- 4 × 100 swim on IHR (focus—hand swapping and stroke count), keep HR below target HR range

IHR

TOTAL YARDAGE: 1,500 yards (includes estimated yards for VK)

COMMENTS

Note this is the first practice in which the shortest distance with no rest is 50 yards rather than 25 yards. Take more rest than indicated or slow down if you are getting out of breath, getting out of your target HR range, or if you feel you need it to execute well. Fast swimming with fins is a great way to notice where you may be offering more resistance than necessary. Faster speeds make turbulence and resistance more noticeable.

SWIMMING GOLF

TOTAL TIME: 30-40 minutes

TARGET HEART RATE RANGE: 70-85% of max heart rate
RPE: 4-7
WARM-UP

- 2 × 50 on :10R—Alt 25 SBDChoice / 25 swim (focus—downhill swimming)
- 2 × 50 on :10R—Alt 25 DBDChoice / 25 swim (focus—side skating)
- 2 × 50 on :10R—Alt 25 SIDChoice / 25 swim (focus—hand/hip connection)
- IHR

WORKOUT

- 4 × 50 SGolf on 2:00 (or 1:00RMin)

IHR
- 3 × 100 on :20RMax SBFins—Alt 25 DChoice / 25 swim (focus—choice)

IHR
- 3 × 50 SGolf on 1:45 (or :45RMin)

IHR
- 1 × 150 SFS FinsOpt

IHR
- 2 × 50 SGolf on 1:30 (or :30RMin)

IHR
Cool-Down
- 6 × 50 on :10R—Alt 25 SGF / 25 5&G

IHR

TOTAL YARDAGE: 1,500 yards

COMMENTS

Expect higher IHRs after SGolf sets. After today's practice, write down your best (lowest) SGolf scores and how you got them—number of strokes, number of seconds, and what you were focusing on to get those scores. In fact, writing down all your SGolf scores in this practice as you do them will come in handy in the Yellow section, when you will repeat these swims for comparison.

7

W
O
R
K
O
U
T

TOTAL TIME: 30-40 minutes

TARGET HEART RATE RANGE: 70-85% of max heart rate

RPE: 4-7

WARM-UP

- 4 × 50 on :10R—Alt 50 SGB Rt / 50 SGB Lft / 50 SFS / 50 swim (focus—side skating)
- 4 × 50 on :10RMax—Alt 25 SGF / 25 swim (focus—hand swapping)
- IHR

WORKOUT

- 3 × 150 on :40R descend 1-3 SBFins—Alt 25 SGB weak / 50 swim (focus—choice) / 25 SGB good / 50 swim (focus—choice)

IHR

- 1 × 200 swim SBFinsOpt (focus—25 side skating / 25 hand swapping)

IHR

- 1 × 100 SGB—Alt 25 Rt / 25 Lft
- 1 × 50 swim (focus—vertical forearm stroke)
- 1 × 50 SGF
- 1 × 50 swim fast (focus—hip snap)

IHR

Cool-Down

- 4 × 75 on :15R—Alt 25 BB / 25 SGBB / 25 SFS

IHR

TOTAL YARDAGE: 1,600 yards

COMMENTS

Longest uninterrupted full-stroke swim yet—200 yards.

FOCUS SWITCHING

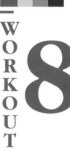

TOTAL TIME: 30-40 minutes

TARGET HEART RATE RANGE: 70-85% of max heart rate
RPE: 4-7
WARM-UP

- 3 × 100 swim Fins on :15RMax (focus—1 side skating, 2 hand swapping, 3 skewer)
- 2 × 100 swim SBFins on :15RMax (focus—1 side skating, 2 downhill swimming)
- 1 × 100 swim (focus—hand/hip connection)
- IHR

WORKOUT

- 10 × 50 on :15RMax—Alt 25 SGB weak / 25 swim fast (focus—odd ones, hip snap; even ones, long reach)

IHR

- 10 × :15 VK on :10R— Dry hands

IHR

Cool-Down

- 6 × 50 on :10R Fins—Alt 25 BBR / 25 SIDChoice

IHR

TOTAL YARDAGE: 1,600 yards (includes estimated yards for VK)

COMMENTS

You should notice less difference between the weak and good sides in those drills where this is an issue. If not, take time to review the drill descriptions from scratch. Have someone else read the description, then watch you execute the drill and give you feedback. Notice the emphasis on switching your focus from one mental image to another.

9

TOTAL TIME: 30-40 minutes

TARGET HEART RATE RANGE: 70-85% of max heart rate

RPE: 4-7

WARM-UP

- 1 × 50 FB
- 1 × 50 BB
- 1 × 50 SGB—Alt 25 Rt / 25 Lft
- 1 × 50 SGBB—Alt 25 Rt / 25 Lft
- 1 × 50 BBR—Alt 25 roll to the Rt / 25 roll to the Lft
- 1 × 50 SFS
- 1 × 50 SGF
- 1 × 50 3&G
- 1 × 50 5&G
- 1 × 50 swim (focus—choice)
- IHR

WORKOUT

- 3 × 100 on :20R—Alt 25 drill / 25 swim (focus—hand swapping and stroke count)
- 3 × 75 on :15RMax—Alt 25 5&G / 25 SFS / 25 5&G
- 3 × 50 on :10RMax—Alt 25 SFS / 25 swim (focus—marionette high elbow recovery)

IHR

- 1 × 25 SGF
- 1 × 25 swim fast (focus—long reach)
- 1 × 25 SGBB weak
- 1 × 25 swim fast (focus—side skating)

IHR

- 1 × 25 SGBB good
- 1 × 25 swim fast (focus—hand swapping)
- 1 × 25 SGF
- 2 × 50 SGolf on 2:00 (or 1:00RMin)

IHR

Cool-Down

- 6 × 50 on :10R—Alt 25 SGB weak / 25 5&G

IHR

TOTAL YARDAGE: 1,750 yards

COMMENTS

It is good to revisit the fundamental drills in progressive order from time to time. How was your experience with these drills today compared with the first time you tried them?

MORE COUNTING

TOTAL TIME: 30-40 minutes

TARGET HEART RATE RANGE: 70-85% of max heart rate
RPE: 4-7
WARM-UP
- 3 × 50 on :10R SBFinsOpt—Alt 25 SGBB weak / 25 5&G
- 3 × 50 on :10R SBFinsOpt—Alt 25 SGBB good / 25 swim (focus—stroke count)
- IHR

WORKOUT

- 4 × 25 swim on :10RMax 1@NS/L, 2@–1S/L, 3@–2S/L, 3@–3S/L

IHR
- 1 × 100 DChoice
- 4 × 50 swim on :20RMax 1@NS/L, 2@–1S/L, 3@–2S/L, 4@–3S/L

IHR
- 1 × 100 DChoice
- 4 × 75 swim on :30RMax 1@NS/L, 2@–1S/L, 3@–2S/L, 4@–3S/L

IHR
- 1 × 100 DChoice
- 4 × :30 VK on :15RMax

IHR
- 3 × 50 SGolf on 1:00RMin

IHR
Cool-Down
- 3 × 100 on :10R FinsOpt—Alt 50 SGBB / 25 SFS / 25 SGF

IHR

TOTAL YARDAGE: 1,800 yards—just over one mile! (includes estimated yardage for VK)

COMMENTS

There is a big emphasis on stroke counting in this practice. You should be looking to lower stroke counts at all speeds. Note that you have to make some choices about which drills to do. Plan ahead. Decide which drill might help you most to accomplish the next swim correctly. Note that because all fin use was optional, you could have done this whole practice with naked feet.

9

Yellow Zone

If you have gone through the Purple zone a couple times and can stay within the Purple target heart rate range most of the time (except when a fast swim or vertical kicking was indicated), it is time to enter the Yellow zone.

Practices in the Yellow zone, like the Purple zone, include from 30- to 50-percent skill drills at moderate intensity. However, these practices will extend into the 40- to 50-minute range, so the total yardage you cover in these practices will be greater than in the Purple zone.

As in the Purple zone, except for using short-blade fins on drills you still need them for, do not use fins unless the practice notation calls for them.

Reading the Workouts

One nice thing about swimming is the ability to incorporate a wide array of physical and mental challenges into any workout. Coaches do this with a variety of cryptic codes that often look more like math homework than a swim workout. With that in mind, allow me to illuminate a few more notations for the coming workouts.

Interval Training

Beginning in the Yellow zone, practices will rely on a format called *interval training*. A training interval is a specified time during which you perform some activity, then rest (for instance, the following set):

4 × 50 swim on 2:00. With this set, you will swim four 50s, beginning every 2 minutes. If it takes you 1:15 to swim the 50, you would get 45 seconds rest after each swim before beginning the next 50. The whole set would take 8 minutes. If it took you only 1:05 to swim the 50, you'd get 55 seconds rest after each 50.

4 × 50 swim on 1:30. If, instead, the set was 4 × 50 swim on 1:30 and it took you 1:15 to swim the 50, you would get only 15 seconds rest after each 50 before starting the next 50, and the whole set would take 6 minutes.

Working With the Pace Clock

With interval training, you will need to become better acquainted with the clock. Because most lap pools have an analog pace clock, the descriptions of how to use the clock will focus on this style of clock. However, the concepts are easily applied to a digital clock, whether it is on the wall or on your wrist.

At first, doing intervals according to the pace clock may seem confusing, but once you've done it a few times you will catch on quickly. Before you move to the Yellow practices, I encourage you to do the following sets to get a better handle on using a pace clock.

4 × 50 swim Fins—Descend 1-4 on 1:15. Swim four 50s with fins on a 1:15 interval, making sure each swim is faster than the previous one. Start the first 50 when the second hand hits the 60 mark. This is referred to as going on the 60. As you finish the swim, note where the second hand is. This tells you how long the swim took. Let's say you finish on the 55 mark. Because the interval is 1:15, swim 2 will leave on the 15 mark (1:15 after the 60 mark where you started the first swim), giving you 20 seconds rest. Try to swim a bit faster. If repeat 2 is the same speed as 1, you would come in on the 10 mark (55 seconds after the 15 mark where swim 2 started). Instead, you swim a 53 (2 seconds faster) and arrive at the wall at the 08 tick mark, between the 5 and 10 numerals. Swim 3 will leave on the 30 mark (1:15 after the 15 mark), so you have 22 seconds rest. Let's say you swim 3 another 2 seconds faster (51 seconds), hitting the wall as the second hand passes the 21-second tick mark. Finally, 4 starts on the 45 mark, you go 50 seconds, your fastest one of the set, and finish as the second hand hits the 35 mark.

Note that the send-off (another name for the time or mark where the next swim begins) for each swim jumps forward on the clock face by 15 seconds—60, 15, 30, 45. If the set had called for five 50s instead of four, the next one would go on the 60 again. If the set had been 4 × 50 swim on 1:10, the send-off would move forward by 10 seconds each repeat—

60, 10, 20, 30. Had the interval been :50, the send-off would move backward on the clock face by 10 seconds for each repeat—60, 50, 40, 30.

When swimming on an interval, the faster you swim the more rest you get before doing the next swim. You may design sets of swims to allow different amounts of rest between swims, depending on the length of each swim. The kind of work you are doing (anaerobic versus aerobic) is determined by the work-to-rest ratio and the intensity of the effort, as shown here.

Various Types of Training				
Type of work	**Work-to-rest ratio**	**Intensity**	**RPE**	**% aerobic vs. anaerobic**
Recovery	3 or more to 1	Low	1-3	95 / 5
Basic endurance	5 or more to 1	Moderate	4-6	90 / 10
Anaerobic threshold	4 or more to 1	High	7-8	80 / 20
Lactate endurance	1 to 1	Very high	8-9	50 / 50
Lactate tolerance	1 to 2 or more	Maximum	9-10	10 / 90

The Yellow section introduces two closely related types of interval training sets, derived directly from your T-swim performances. Each time you complete a T-swim, you use the Cruise Pace per 100 Chart in appendix A to determine the average pace per 100 you maintained during the T-swim. Once you know your cruise pace, it is easy to use two other charts—the Cruise Interval Chart in appendix C and the Cruise Times Chart in appendix B—to determine proper aerobic and anaerobic threshold training paces for various distances.

Cruise Pace and Cruise Times

The Cruise Times Chart in appendix B shows how long it takes to swim various distances, from 25 up to 500 at any cruise pace. Simply locate your cruise pace per 100 in the column and look across that row for cruise times at different distances. You'll begin to see sets using information from the Cruise Times Chart:

11-minute set, swim 200s @ CPace on :10 to :15R. This example asks you to swim an 11-minute set of 200s at your cruise pace (let's say it is 1:37 per 100), and take between 10 and 15 seconds rest after each one. Locate 1:37 in the Cruise Pace per 100 column on the Cruise Times Chart and look across to the CT200 column. The entry there is 3:14. If you swim at your cruise pace you'll hit 3:14. Leaving on the 3:25 for the next swim gives you between 10 and 15 seconds rest. The fourth one in the set would begin at 10:15. Because the 11-minute period is not yet complete, you start the swim and complete the lap that the 11-minute mark falls in. Sets designed around cruise pace with added short rests are excellent aerobic basic endurance training and are not overly stressful because of the added rest.

Cruise Intervals

Once you know your cruise pace, it is easy to determine proper and challenging anaerobic threshold (fastest pace you can maintain for an extended time) training intervals for various distances. These intervals, based on your cruise pace, are called cruise intervals. Each cruise interval entry in appendix C indicates both an interval and a target time to hit or beat on each swim. A section of appendix C is shown here.

Cruise Intervals					
CPace (per 100)	Cruise interval				
	25	50	100	150	200
⋮					
⋮					
1:49	:35-26	1:00-53	2:00-45	2:55-42	3:55-34
1:48	:35-26	1:00-52	2:00-44	2:55-38	3:50-35
1:47	:35-25	1:00-51	1:55-45	2:55-36	3:50-30

A cruise interval set might look like this.

12-minute set, swim 200s on CInt. Say the cruise pace per 100 you looked up after your most recent T-swim is 1:48, and you want to know what your cruise interval for 200-yard swims is.

1. Find 1:48 in the CPace per 100 column.

2. Look across the 1:48 line to the CInt200 (cruise interval 200) column.

3. The entry in the CInt200 column is 3:50-35. This means your interval is 3:50 and your target time to hit or beat on every swim is 3:35. This will give you about 15 seconds rest before the next swim starts. (Note that the CInt100 entry on this same line—2:00-44—means an interval of 2:00 and a target time of 1:44, not 2:44.)

4. Because your interval is 3:50, you'll have time to complete four full repeats and a portion of repeat number five. Always swim through the entire set duration, finishing the lap that the 12 minute falls on at the same pace as the rest of the swim (or faster).

Cruise intervals and their target times are calculated to be challenging but doable. As you have T-swim improvements, you may find that hitting your new target time on the interval is hard to do for more than a few repeats. That's OK. The idea behind cruise intervals is to get outside your comfort zone, but not outside of your near-term improvement possibilities.

Last One Fast One

On cruise pace and cruise interval sets, you will often see LOFO in the set description. This means that you are to swim the last repeat significantly faster than the preceding repeats. Where you see LOFO, it is OK to take up to three times the amount of rest that the interval has allowed for the other swims in the set.

New Focus Point

To keep the learning and refining process in gear, here is another concept to tickle your gray matter while you are wet:

- **Surge and skate:** As you drill and swim, with every stroke there is a period when you feel yourself surge forward in the water and a period when you are skating along on one side, preparing to take the next stroke. I liken this to a speed skater—each time he shifts his weight onto one skate as he pushes off with the other skate, there is a noticeable surge of speed (this correlates to our roll of the body and the stroke you take during that roll). After the weight shift, there is a period of sliding with no propulsion as he prepares to make the next weight shift (this correlates to our streamlined side-lying position, as the recovering arm is moving forward toward the point where it will again enter the water). In swimming, the surge is greatest when we maintain the hand and hip connection, and the skating action is most effective when we have a balanced, streamlined position, allowing maximum conservation of speed.

Moving right along, now that you are primed with new training and technique concepts, let's move on to the Yellow practices. Before you do, though, turn to the appendix and copy down two sets of numbers for quick reference. On the Cruise Times Chart, copy down the row of times and associated distances for your most recent cruise pace per 100. On the Cruise Interval Chart, find your cruise pace per 100 and copy the row of cruise intervals and target times for each distance across the chart. Put these in a zipper sandwich bag to use on deck during your practice sessions. Now get yourself to the pool.

TOTAL TIME: 40-50 minutes

TARGET HEART RATE RANGE: 70-85% of max heart rate
RPE: 4-7
WARM-UP
- 4 × 25 on :10R SBFinsOpt— Alt 25 DChoice / 25 swim
- 4 × 50 3&G on :10RMax
- IHR

WORKOUT

- 4 × 25 swim on :10R (focus—hand/hip connection) descend 1-4
- 8-minute set, swim CPace 50s on :10 to :15R (focus—odd ones, downhill swimming; even ones, long reach)

IHR
- 1 × 150 SBFinsOpt—Alt 50 3&G / 50 5&G / 50 swim (focus—surge and skate)
- 4 × 50 on :15R—Alt 25 3&G / 25 swim (focus—stroke count, odd ones @NS/L, even ones @–2S/L)

IHR
- 1 × 4-minute CPace swim (shortest distance in which cruise pace exceeds 4:00)

IHR
- 3 × 100 on :20RMax—Alt 25 SGBB weak / swim 25 (focus—skewer) / 25 SGBB good / swim 25 (focus—skewer)

IHR
Cool-Down
- 2 × 25 swim on :15RMax (focus—side skating) 1@NS/L, 1@–2S/L
- 4 × 25 on :15RMax FinsOpt—Alt 25 FB / 25 SGB Lft / 25 BB / 25 SGB Rt
- 2 × 25 swim on :15R (focus—downhill swimming) both @–1S/L

IHR

TOTAL YARDAGE: approximately 1,800 yards

COMMENTS

If you would like to do some cruise pace and cruise interval sets with fins, then you will need to do a T-swim with fins so you'll have an appropriate set of times to work with. Throughout the remainder of the practices, total yardage will be approximated for a person with a cruise pace of 1:50 per 100. Faster swimmers will rack up more yardage and slower swimmers less.

2 WORKOUT

TOTAL TIME: 40-50 minutes

TARGET HEART RATE RANGE: 70-85% of max heart rate

RPE: 4-7

WARM-UP

- 4 × 25 on :10RMax FinsOpt—Alt 25 FB / 25 3&G
- 4 × 25 on :10RMax SBFins—Alt 25 SGB Rt / 25 SGBB Rt / 25 SGB Lft / 25 SGBB Lft
- 4 × 25 on :10R—Alt 25 SGB good / 25 swim (focus—downhill swimming)
- IHR

WORKOUT

- 8 × 25 on :15RMax—Alt 25 FB / 25 SGB good / 25 BB / 25 swim (focus—stroke count)

IHR

- 4 × :15 VK on :10R—Hands on your chest

IHR

- 6 × 75 on :10RMax SBFinsOpt—Alt 25 FB / 25 SGB weak / 25 swim (focus—surge and skate)
- 6-minute set, swim 50s at CPace on :5 to :10R LOFO

IHR

- 6 × :15 VK SBFins on :10R—Dry hands

IHR

- 6-minute set, swim 50s on CInt

IHR

- 6 × :15 VK Fins on :10R—Dry elbows and hands

IHR

Cool-Down

- 2 × 100 on :15RMax—Alt 25 SGBB weak / 25 swim (focus—stroke count and hand swapping)

TOTAL YARDAGE: approximately 1,950 yards (includes estimated yards for VK)

You can see the difference between a CPace set and a CInt set. So far these sets have been short. As the workouts progress, the duration of these sets will increase to make them more aerobic. Be sure to move from one line of the practice to the next as quickly as possible so your heart rate doesn't get below the 120 to 130 range.

TOTAL TIME: 40-50 minutes

TARGET HEART RATE RANGE: 70-85% of max heart rate
RPE: 4-7
WARM-UP

- 8 × 25 on :15RMax FinsOpt—Alt 25 FB / 25 SGB Rt / 25 BB / 25 SGB Lft
- 2 × 75 swim on :20R (focus—25 long reach / 25 marionette high elbow recovery / 25 laser beam body-roll trigger)
- IHR

WORKOUT

- 10 × 25 on :15RMax—Alt 25 3&G / 25 swim (focus—stroke count; don't let the S/L go up as the set progresses)

IHR

- 5 × 50 on :15RMax—Alt 25 5&G / 25 swim (focus—hand and hip connection)

IHR

- 8 × :15 VK SBFins on :15R—Odd ones, hands on your chest; even ones, dry hands and elbows

IHR

- 6-minute set, swim 100s @ CPace on :10 to :15R (focus—stroke count; don't let it go up)

IHR

- 6-minute set, swim 50s on CInt (focus—hip snap) LOFO

IHR
Cool-Down

- 6 × 25 swim on :10R (focus—downhill swimming) 2@NS/L, 2@–2S/L, 2@–3S/L
- 4 × 50 DChoice SBFins on :10R

IHR

TOTAL YARDAGE: approximately 1,950 yards (includes estimated yards for VK)

COMMENTS

Going from the CPace set to the CInt set may be challenging. Try to keep the same stroke count per length throughout both sets.

WORKOUT 4

TOTAL TIME: 40-50 minutes

TARGET HEART RATE RANGE: 70-85% of max heart rate
RPE: 4-7
WARM-UP

- 4 × 25 on :10R Fins—Alt 25 BBR / 25 SGBB Rt / 25 BBR / 25 SGBB Lft
- 4 × 25 on :10R SBFins—Alt 25 BBR / 25 SGBB Rt / 25 BBR / 25 SGBB Lft
- 4 × 25 on :10R—Alt 25 BBR / 25 SGBB Rt / 25 BBR / 25 SGBB Lft
- 1 × 100—Alt 25 SGBB / 25 swim (focus—surge and skate)
- IHR

WORKOUT

- 8-minute set, swim 50s (focus—stroke count) on IHR (HR in target range)
- 1 × 50 SFS
- 1 × 50 SGBB—Alt 25 Rt / 25 Lft
IHR
- 8-minute set, swim 50s on CInt LOFO (focus—odd ones, hand and hip connection; even ones hip snap)
- 1 × 50 SFS (focus—hand/hip connection)
- 1 × 50 5&G (focus—vertical forearm stroke)
IHR
- 6 × :20 VK on :15R—Odd ones, hands on chest; even ones, dry hands
IHR
- 1 × 4:00 swim @ CPace
Cool-Down
- 4 × 75 on :15RMax SBFins—Alt 25 SGBB /25 SFS / 25 3&G
IHR

TOTAL YARDAGE: approximately 2,000 yards (includes estimated yards for VK)

COMMENTS

Always take some aspect of a drill you have mastered and duplicate it in your full-stroke swimming. Are you getting more comfortable with CPace and CInt swims? On CInt sets it is OK to swim faster than the target time indicated on the chart on some repeats, but only if none of them are slower than the target time.

TOTAL TIME: 40-50 minutes

TARGET HEART RATE RANGE: 70-85% of max heart rate

RPE: 4-7

WARM-UP

- 6 × 75 on :15R SBFins—Alt 25 SGBB Rt / 25 SGBB Lft / 25 swim (focus—skewer)
- IHR

WORKOUT

- 6 × 50 on :15RMax—Alt 50 SFS / 50 SGF / 50 3&G

IHR

- 6 × 50 on :15R Fins—Alt 25 3&G / 25 swim fast (focus—surge and skate)

IHR

- 8 × :20 VK on :10R—Odd ones, dry hands; even ones, dry hands and elbows

IHR

- 10-minute set, swim 100s @ CPace on :10 to :15R (focus—stroke count) LOFO

Cool-Down

- 4 × 100 5&G on IHR (focus—hand swapping), keep HR below target HR range

TOTAL YARDAGE: approximately 2,100 yards (includes estimated yards for VK)

COMMENTS

Fast swimming with fins is a great way to notice where you may be offering more resistance than necessary. The CPace set indicated you should swim last one fast one—were you able to avoid adding strokes?

6

TOTAL TIME: 40-50 minutes

TARGET HEART RATE RANGE: 70-85% of max heart rate

RPE: 4-7

WARM-UP

- 2 × 50 on :10R—Alt 25 SBDChoice / 25 SFS
- 2 × 50 on :10R—Alt 25 DBDChoice / 25 swim (focus—surge and skate)
- 2 × 50 on :10R—Alt 25 SIDChoice / 25 swim (focus—hand swapping)
- IHR

WORKOUT

- 4 × 50 SGolf on 2:00 (or 1:00RMin)

IHR

- 3 × 100 on :20RMax SBFins—Alt 25 DChoice / 25 3&G

IHR

- 3 × 50 SGolf on 1:45 (or :45RMin)

IHR

- 1 × 150 SFS FinsOpt (focus—vertical forearm stroke)

IHR

- 2 × 50 SGolf on 1:30 (or :30RMin)

IHR

- 12-minute set, swim 100s on CInt LOFO

Cool-Down

- 6 × 50 on :10R—Alt 25 SGB / 25 5&G (focus—hand/hip connection)

IHR

TOTAL YARDAGE: approximately 2,100 yards

Compare your swimming golf (SGolf) scores with the ones you wrote down after Purple practice 6. Because this practice is the same as that practice (until you come to the 12-minute CInt set after the SGolf swims), you will be comparing apples to apples.

TOTAL TIME: 40-50 minutes

TARGET HEART RATE RANGE: 70-85% of max heart rate
RPE: 4-7
WARM-UP

- 4 × 50 on :10R—Alt 50 SGB Rt / 50 SGB Lft / 50 SFS / 50 swim (focus—surge and skate)
- 4 × 50 on :10RMax—Alt 25 SGF / 25 swim (focus—hand swapping)
- IHR

WORKOUT

- 3 × 100 on :40R descend 1-3 SBFins—Alt 25 SGB weak / 25 swim (focus—choice) / 25 SGB good / 25 swim (focus—choice)

IHR

- 1 × 200 swim SBFinsOpt (focus—hand/hip connection)

IHR

- 1 × 100 SGB—Alt 25 Rt / 25 Lft
- 1 × 50 swim fast (focus—downhill swimming)
- 1 × 50 SGF
- 1 × 50 swim fast Fins (focus—hip snap)

IHR

- 15-minute set, swim 200s @ CPace on :20 to :30R (focus—50 downhill swimming, 50 long reach, 50 hand swapping, 50 hand/hip connection)

IHR
Cool-Down

- 4 × 75 on :15R—Alt 25 BB / 25 SGBB / 25 SFS

IHR

TOTAL YARDAGE: approximately 2,200 yards

Longest CPace set yet—changing your focus points regularly will help keep you on track with technique and pass the time quickly.

W
O
R
K
O
U
T

8

TOTAL TIME: 40-50 minutes

TARGET HEART RATE RANGE: 70-85% of max heart rate

RPE: 4-7

WARM-UP

- 3 × 100 swim Fins on :15RMax (focus—1 surge and skate, 2 hand swapping, 3 skewer)
- 2 × 100 swim SBFins on :15RMax (focus—1 surge and skate, 2 downhill swimming)
- 1 × 100 swim (focus—downhill swimming)
- IHR

WORKOUT

- 20 × 50 on :10R—Odd ones, SGB 25 weak / 25 good; even ones, swim 50 @ CPace (focus—long reach)

IHR

- 1 × 100 swim—In how few strokes can you do the whole 100?

IHR

- 10 × :15 VK on :10R— Dry hands

IHR

Cool-Down

- 6 × 50 on :10R Fins—Alt 25 BBR / 25 SIDChoice

IHR

TOTAL YARDAGE: approximately 2,200 yards (includes estimated yards for VK)

COMMENTS

As you are doing that set of 20 × 50, alternating between drill and CPace swimming, keep the drill going at a fast enough pace so that your heart rate doesn't go down much. By the way, did you have to look up your CPace time for 50s or did you remember it? Eventually you will be familiar with most of your shorter CPace times.

TOTAL TIME: 40-50 minutes

TARGET HEART RATE RANGE: 70-85% of max heart rate
RPE: 4-7
WARM-UP

- 1 × 100 Alt 50 FB/50 BB
- 1 × 50 SGB—Alt 25 Rt / 25 Lft
- 1 × 50 SGBB—weak side
- 1 × 50 BBR—Alt 25 roll 360s to the Rt / 25 roll 360s to the Lft
- 1 × 100 Alt 50 SFS/50 SGF
- 1 × 100 3&G
- 1 × 50 swim (focus—choice)
- IHR

WORKOUT

- 2 × 100 on :20R—Alt 25Choice / 25 swim (focus—hand swapping and stroke count)
- 2 × 75 on :15RMax—Alt 25 5&G / 25 SFS / 25 5&G
- 2 × 50 on :10RMax—Alt 25 SFS / 25 swim (focus—marionette high elbow recovery)
- 2 × 25 on :5R—Swim for fewest strokes possible

IHR
- 1 × 50 Alt 25 SGF (focus—vertical forearm stroke)/25 swim fast (focus—stroke count)
- 1 × 50 Alt 25 SGBB weak/25 swim fast (focus—surge and skate)
- 1 × 50 SGBB good/25 SGF (focus—hand/hip connection)
- 6 × 25 swim fast fins (focus—long reach and hip snap) on :30RMax

IHR
- 15-minute set, swim choice of 100s or 150s or 200s on CInt (focus—pick two and alternate them between each swim) LOFO

IHR
Cool-Down
- 6 × 50 on :10R—Alt 25 SGB weak / 25 5&G

IHR

TOTAL YARDAGE: approximately 2,300 yards

Revisiting the fundamental drills in progressive order is an excellent way to spend time in a pool that is not conducive to normal practices. That set of fast 25s with fins on longer than normal rest may get your heart rate out of target range.

10

TOTAL TIME: 40-50 minutes

TARGET HEART RATE RANGE: 70-85% of max heart rate

RPE: 4-7

WARM-UP

- 3 × 50 on :10R—Alt 25 SGBB weak / 25 5&G
- 3 × 50 on :10R—Alt 25 SGBB good / 25 swim (focus—stroke count)
- IHR

WORKOUT

- 5-minute set, swim 25s CInt—Alt 2@NS/L, 2@–1S/L LOFO

IHR

- 1 × 100 DChoice FinsOpt
- 7-minute set, swim 50s CInt—Alt 2@NS/L, 2@–1S/L LOFO

IHR

- 1 × 100 DChoice
- 9-minute set, swim 75s CInt—Alt 1@NS/L, 1@–1S/L LOFO

IHR

- 1 × 100 DChoice FinsOpt
- 4 × :30 VK on :15RMax

IHR

- 3 × 50 SGB fast on :30RMax

IHR

Cool-Down

- 3 × 100 on :10R—Alt 50 SGBB / 25 SFS / 25 SGF

IHR

TOTAL YARDAGE: approximately 2,300 yards (includes estimated yardage for VK)

COMMENTS

There is a big emphasis on stroke counting while keeping speed on target. You should lower stroke counts at all speeds. Plan ahead for which drill might help you most to accomplish the next swim correctly. The fast SGB set shows that you can use drills as high-intensity training too, but strict attention to proper execution and feedback points is still vital!

10

Orange Zone

The moderate intensity practices in the Yellow zone included up to 50-percent skill drills. As you move into the Orange zone there will be less drilling and more swimming. Yet, the focus will still be technique oriented, rather than slogging out yardage. Each Orange practice involves either one highly anaerobic set (very fast swimming with moderate to long rest) or a large amount of cruise interval work. Attempt the practices in the Orange zone only after you've been doing the practices in the Purple and Yellow zones long enough to be comfortable with them. You should, by this time, have mastered all the drills.

Speed Training

In the Yellow zone, I introduced the concept of cruise intervals to improve endurance at the highest aerobic speeds. The Orange zone introduces three new types of sets specifically for developing higher, more anaerobic speeds. Short sprint sets develop maximum, short-term, explosive speed. Lactate endurance and lactate tolerance sets improve pain tolerance and your body's ability to deal with lactic acid accumulation while swimming fast. These last two types of sets require maximum efforts and maximum or near-maximum speeds. I offer them as test sets, to motivate you to do them at the appropriate intensity.

Reading the Workouts

The notation for these new types of sets may require close attention the first few times you see them.

Short Sprint Sets

You have already seen a few places where you are to do short repeats, fast. Let's expand that:

6 × 25 swim AFAP OACI. This type of set calls for very fast swimming with lots of rest. This set notation asks you to swim 6 × 25 as fast as possible (AFAP) on any comfortable interval (OACI). Comfortable interval means long enough to allow enough rest (or easy swim and drill), so you can swim the next one fast without fatigue or pain. The amount of rest needed will vary from person to person. If in doubt, err on the side of too much rather than too little rest. If a full length of the pool takes you more than 15 seconds, you should sprint only a portion of the length, perhaps three-fourths or one-half the length. This type of set of very short, fast swims trains the anaerobic alactic (does not accumulate lactic acid) system.

Test Sets

From the beginning you have been doing T-swims and recording your results. This is referred to as a *test set*—a set that you repeat from time to time, recording your results each time (see chapter 14 for charts). The idea is, over time, to see improvements in your technique, speed, and endurance. Orange practices introduce two new types of test sets: lactate endurance sets and lactate tolerance sets.

In the set notation, the word TEST precedes all test sets. In addition to showing what to swim, each set will ask for specific information, indicated in brackets (i.e., [fast2, slow, avgS/L] indicates that you are to record the times of the two fastest swims, the time of the slowest swim, and your average number of strokes per length).

Lactate Endurance Sets

Lactate endurance (LE) sets call for swimming high-intensity repeats on roughly a 1:1 work-to-rest ratio. This allows enough rest to recover partially but not completely between repeats. This type of set produces increasing lactic acid levels and high heart rates throughout the set. This improves your ability to perform consistently for an extended time at high speeds, despite a high level of lactic acid. It also improves your body's ability to buffer lactic acid.

During a set of this nature, in which you are getting a fair amount of rest, you should keep moving (drills, easy swimming, bobbing, etc.) to speed recovery. This is referred to as *active rest*. In some cases the set notation will suggest a specific activity.

LACTATE ENDURANCE TEST

1. 16-minute set, swim 50s on 1:1 W/RInt; :02Range
   [interval, fast2, slow, avgS/L]

This notation calls for a 16-minute set of very fast 50s on a 1:1 work-to-rest ratio interval—meaning that the rest period between swims should be roughly the same length as the work period. If each swim takes you about 34 seconds, then your interval would be 1:10. This allows 36 seconds rest, roughly 1:1 work-to-rest ratio. If your average swim time in this set is 32, then 1:05 would be a more appropriate interval. If in doubt, choose the interval that gives slightly less rest. The :02Range means you should allow no more than two seconds difference between the speeds of the slowest and fastest swims in the set. At the end of this set, record the interval that you were swimming on, the times of the two fastest swims, the time of the slowest swim, and your average number of strokes per length. (It is not necessary to count your strokes every length of the swim. Count strokes on 8 to 10 lengths, spaced evenly across the set duration, excluding the first length of any repeat.) Test sets for 75s, 100s, and 200s have similar notation:

ADDITIONAL LACTATE ENDURANCE TEST SETS

2. 18-minute set, swim 75s on 1:1 W/RInt; :03Range
   [interval, fast2, slow, avgS/L]
3. 20-minute set, swim 100s on 1:1 W/RInt; :04Range
   [interval, fast2, slow, avgS/L]
4. 24-minute set, swim 200s on 1:1 W/RInt; :06Range
   [interval, fast2, slow, avgS/L]

If your interval allows you to start the next repetition before the end of the allotted time, then do so and swim the whole distance.

Lactate Tolerance Sets

Lactate tolerance (LT) sets improve your body's ability to buffer the effects of high levels of lactic acid. You do this with repeated swims at maximum or near-maximum speeds, with long rests between them. The longer rests allow more recovery from one swim to the next than during LE sets. Because of this, the swimming speeds should be faster, the lactic acid levels will be higher, and, consequently, these sets are more painful than LE sets.

LACTATE TOLERANCE TEST

1. Swim 4 × 100 (or 75, 2:00Cut) on 6:00 w/50s EZ drill and swim mix on IHR
   [fast2, slow, avgS/L]

This set notation asks for 4 all-out 100s on a 6-minute interval with however much easy recovery swimming and drilling (active rest) you have time for between each. The 2:00Cut means that if you can't finish 100 under 2:00, then you should opt for 75s instead. Record the two fastest swims and the slowest swim as well as the average strokes per length. When doing the EZ drill and swim stuff between the repeats of fast swimming, check your heart rate often. The idea is to let it come down to near the bottom of your GATHRR (general aerobic training heart rate range) and hold it there. Because you'll get anywhere from two to five times as much rest as work, this set is highly anaerobic in nature. LT sets for 50s and 200s use similar notation:

ADDITIONAL LACTATE TOLERANCE TEST SETS

2. Swim 8 × 50 on 3:00 (or 6 on 4:00, 1:00Cut) w/25s EZ drill and swim mix on IHR
   [fast2, slow, avgS/L]
3. Swim 3 × 200 (or 150, 4:00Cut) on 12:00 w/100s EZ drill and swim mix on IHR
   [fast2, slow, avgS/L]

On the set of eight 50s, if you can't make the 1:00 cut, go 6 × 50 on the longer interval rather than dropping to a shorter distance. On the shorter distance sets (50s and 100s), it is an excellent idea to have someone else timing you with a stopwatch to get precise times. Otherwise, you may miss speed improvements that come in fractions of seconds if you are timing yourself on a pace clock.

Frequency of High-Stress Training

Lactate endurance and lactate tolerance training sets are stressful, and only well-conditioned swimmers can tolerate them two or three times per week. Don't do this type of training on back-to-back days. By the time you graduate to doing workouts in the Orange and Red zones, you should be following one of the training programs in chapter 13.

New Focus Point

Once you have digested this information on new training sets, your brain may still be hungry for a new technique idea (think of it as dessert).

- **Hip rhythm:** Our technique uses hip and torso rotation as the engine of propulsion, relying on the shoulders, arms, and hands as the transmission linking our power source to the water. As we increase swimming speed, we want to do it by increasing stroke rate without giving up stroke length. Therefore, the rhythm of freestyle swimming must increase at the hips rather than at the arms and shoulders. If you want to go faster, you should do it by getting from one side-skating position to the next side-skating position, then back to the first more rapidly, while maintaining the hand and hip connection. If, instead, you just move your arms faster, you will lose the hand and hip connection and the surge of speed that body roll could provide. Set your swimming rhythm at your hips, not at your shoulders.

Now that you are primed with new training and technique concepts, let's move to the Orange practices. Do not use fins unless the practice notation calls for them, with two exceptions: (1) Cruise pace and cruise interval sets—if you have done a T-swim with fins, then it is OK to do CPace and CInt sets, in moderation, with fins; (2) Lactate endurance and tolerance sets—once you have done each test set with no fins, you may do some with short-blade fins for more variety. Record these results separately from your naked test sets.

**W
O
R
K
O
U
T**

1

TOTAL TIME: 40-50 minutes

TARGET HEART RATE RANGE: 75-90% of max heart rate

RPE: 7-9

WARM-UP

10-minute set:

- 1 × 25 FB
- 1 × 25 BB
- 1 × 50 SGB—Alt 25 Rt / 25 Lft
- 1 × 50 SGBB—Alt 25 Rt / 25 Lft
- 1 × 50 BBR—Alt 25 roll 360s to the Rt / 25 roll 360s to the Lft
- 1 × 25 SFS

- 1 × 25 SGF
- 1 × 25 3&G
- 1 × 25 5&G
- 50s swim (focus— choice) descending on :10R to finish 10 minutes
- IHR

WORKOUT

- 16-minute set, swim 250s (or 200s or 150s) on CInt (focus—stroke count; take one less stroke on the last length of each repeat)

IHR

- 5-minute set, fast 25s Fins on :10RMax—Alt 25 swim (focus—hip rhythm) / 25 kick

IHR

- 10-minute set, swim 100s (or 50s) on CInt LOFO (focus—pick two and alternate each swim)

IHR

Cool-Down

- 8-minute set, continuous swim starting at CPace and gradually getting slower while decreasing stroke count throughout the swim

IHR

TOTAL YARDAGE: assuming 1:20/100 cruise pace, approximately 3,000 yards; assuming 1:40/100 cruise pace, approximately 2,400 yards; assuming 2:00/100 cruise pace, approximately 2,000 yards

COMMENTS

We revisit the fundamental drills in progressive order. Try to do the whole progression without stopping. In the main set, there is no extra rest other than what you need for taking heart rates and making equipment changes.

TOTAL TIME: 40-50 minutes

TARGET HEART RATE RANGE: 75-90% of max heart rate
RPE: 7-9
WARM-UP

- 4 × 25 on :10RMax SBFins—Alt 25 SGB Rt / 25 SGBB Rt / 25 SGB Lft / 25 SGBB Lft
- 4 × 25 on :10R—Alt 25 SGB good / 25 swim (focus—downhill swimming)
- 6-minute set, 75s on :10RMax SBFinsOpt—Alt 25 FB / 25 SGB weak / 25 swim (focus—surge and skate)
- 6-minute set, swim 50s at CPace on :5 to :10R
- IHR

WORKOUT

- 6 × 25 swim AFAP OACI

IHR

- 20-minute set, swim 300s (or any longer distance) on CInt LOFO

IHR

Cool-Down

- 8-minute set, 100s on :10RMax FinsOpt—Alt 25 SGBB / 25 swim (focus—surge and skate, hand swapping)

TOTAL YARDAGE: assuming 1:20/100 cruise pace, approximately 2,350 yards; assuming 1:40/100 cruise pace, approximately 1,900 yards; assuming 2:00/100 cruise pace, approximately 1,600 yards

COMMENTS

On the 20-minute cruise interval set, it's OK to choose a different distance for the last repeat of the set so your finish time is near 20 minutes. If you decided to go 400s and your CInt is 7:45, your third repeat would start at 15:30 and end at 23:15. You might, instead, choose to swim a 250—CInt 4:50—on the last repeat, which would allow you to finish the set at 20:20, much closer to the intended set duration.

3

TOTAL TIME: 40-50 minutes

TARGET HEART RATE RANGE: 75-90% of max heart rate
RPE: 7-9
WARM-UP

- 4-minute set, drill 50s on :10R—Alt 25 SGBB weak / 25 SGF
- 4-minute set, drill and swim FinsOpt 50s on :10R—Alt 25 SGBB weak / 25 swim (focus—stroke count)
- 4-minute set, swim SBFinsOpt 25s for lowest stroke count on :10R
- IHR

WORKOUT

- 14-minute set, swim 300s (or 250s or 200s) on CInt
IHR
- 10-minute set, swim 100s (or 75s or 50s) on CInt
IHR
- 6-minute set, swim @ CPace (choose shortest chart distance with cruise time of 6:00 or longer, and try to hit your cruise time on the nose)
IHR
Cool-Down
- 6-minute set, 100s on :10R—Alt 25 SGBB / 25 SGF/ 50 swim (focus—hip rhythm)
IHR

TOTAL YARDAGE: assuming 1:20/100 cruise pace, approximately 2,850 yards; assuming 1:40/100 cruise pace, approximately 2,300 yards; assuming 2:00/100 cruise pace, approximately 1,900 yards

COMMENTS

During the main set, there is no extra rest between sets. Also, try to get a lower stroke count on the last length of each repeat in the cruise interval sets.

TOTAL TIME: 40-50 minutes

TARGET HEART RATE RANGE: 75-100% of max heart rate
RPE: 7-10
WARM-UP

- 12-minute continuous drill and swim—Alt 25 SFS / 75 swim (focus—25 long reach / 25 laser beam body-roll trigger / 25 stroke count)
- IHR

WORKOUT

- 6-minute set, 75s on :10RMax FinsOpt —Alt 25 swim AFAP (focus—hip rhythm) / 50 SGBB

IHR

- TEST (LE), 16-minute set, swim 50s on 1:1 W/RInt :02Range [interval, fast2, slow, avgS/L]

IHR

- 6-minute set, swim 50s on CPace on :10 to :15R LOFO (focus—stroke count; don't let it go up)

IHR
Cool-Down

- 4-minute set, 100s on :10RMax Fins—Alt 25 BBR / 25 SGBB Rt / 25 BBR / 25 SGBB Lft

IHR

- 4-minute set, 50s DChoice SBFins on :10R

IHR

TOTAL YARDAGE: assuming 1:20/100 cruise pace, approximately 2,350 yards; assuming 1:40/100 cruise pace, approximately 1,900 yards; assuming 2:00/100 cruise pace, approximately 1,600 yards

COMMENTS

Going from the test set to the CPace set may be challenging. You should be able to keep a lower stroke count during the CPace set than during the test set.

5

TOTAL TIME: 40-50 minutes

TARGET HEART RATE RANGE: 75-100% of max heart rate

RPE: 7-10

WARM-UP

- 12-minute set, swim 50s (focus—stroke count; don't let it go up) on IHR, start slow and gradually increase intensity so HR moves from bottom of GATHRR to top of GATHRR

WORKOUT

- TEST (LE), 18-minute set, swim 75s on 1:1 W/RInt :03Range [interval, fast2, slow, avgS/L] (perhaps go an EZ 50 of SGF during the rest between each fast 75)

IHR

- 2 × 50 EZ on :10R—Alt 25 SFS / 25 SGF

IHR

- 8-minute set, swim 100s on CInt (focus—stroke count, surge and skate) LOFO

IHR

Cool-Down

- 8-minute set, 100s FinsOpt 5&G on IHR (focus—hand swapping), keep HR near bottom of GATHRR

TOTAL YARDAGE: assuming 1:20/100 cruise pace, approximately 2,650 yards; assuming 1:40/100 cruise pace, approximately 2,100 yards; assuming 2:00/100 cruise pace, approximately 1,750 yards

COMMENTS

Start the warm-up slower than you think you need to. Move from one item of the main set to the next with no extra rest—just check your HR and go. LOFO means last one fast one—staying on your interval, try to swim the last repeat of the set significantly faster than the others.

TOTAL TIME: 40-50 minutes

TARGET HEART RATE RANGE: 75-100% of max heart rate

RPE: 7-10

WARM-UP

12-minute set:

- 2 × 50 on :10R—Alt 25 SBDChoice / 25 SFS
- 2 × 50 on :10R—Alt 25 DBDChoice / 25 swim (focus—surge and skate)
- 2 × 50 on :10R—Alt 25 SIDChoice / 25 swim (focus—hand swapping)
- 50s swim (focus—stroke count) on :10R to finish the 12 minutes
- IHR

WORKOUT

- 3 × 50 SGolf on :45RMax (focus—hip rhythm)

IHR

- TEST (LE), 20-minute set, swim 100s on 1:1 W/RInt :04Range [interval, fast2, slow, avgS/L] (perhaps go an EZ 75 or 50 of SGF or SGBB during the rest between each fast 100)

IHR

- 3 × 50 SGolf on :30RMax

IHR

Cool-Down

- 8-minute set, swim 100s on CInt (just make the interval)

IHR

TOTAL YARDAGE: assuming 1:20/100 cruise pace, approximately 2,650 yards; assuming 1:40/100 cruise pace, approximately 2,150 yards; assuming 2:00/100 cruise pace, approximately 1,750 yards

COMMENTS

Try to keep your scores in the second set of SGolf at or below your scores in the first SGolf set. During the cool-down, instead of trying to meet or beat the target time on the CInt chart, just swim fast enough to barely make the interval.

**W
O
R
K
O
U
T**

7

TOTAL TIME: 40-50 minutes

TARGET HEART RATE RANGE: 75-100% of max heart rate
RPE: 7-10
WARM-UP
10-minute set:

- 2 × 100 (or 75 or 50) swim Fins on IHR (focus—surge and skate)
- 2 × 100 (or 75 or 50) swim SBFins on IHR (focus—downhill swimming)
- 2 × 100 (or 75 or 50) swim (focus—hand swapping) on IHR
- 25s swim on :5 to :10R descending to finish 10-minute set
- IHR

WORKOUT

- TEST (LE), 24-minute set, swim 200s on 1:1 W/RInt :06Range [interval, fast2, slow, avgS/L] (perhaps alternating 25 swim (low stroke count) and 25 SGB between fast 200s)

IHR

- 1 × 100 EZ swim—In how few strokes can you do the whole 100?

IHR

- 1 × 100 swim—How fast can you go without using more strokes to swim the 100?

IHR
Cool-Down

- 8-minute set, 6 × 50 on :10R Fins—Alt 25 BBR / 25 SIDChoice
- EZ 50s swim on :5 to :10R (focus—hand swapping) to finish 8 minutes

IHR

TOTAL YARDAGE: assuming 1:20/100 cruise pace, approximately 2,650 yards; assuming 1:40/100 cruise pace, approximately 2,100 yards; assuming 2:00/100 cruise pace, approximately 1,750 yards

COMMENTS

If your interval allows you to start the last 200 anytime before the 24-minute mark, go ahead and swim the whole distance, even though it takes you past 24 minutes.

LACTATE TOLERANCE #1

TOTAL TIME: 40-50 minutes

TARGET HEART RATE RANGE: 75-100% of max heart rate
RPE: 7-10
WARM-UP

- 6-minute set, SBFinsOpt 100s on :10RMax—Alt 25 DChoice / 50 3&G / 25 swim
- 8-minute set, swim CPace 50s on :10 to :15R (focus—odd ones, downhill swimming; even ones, long reach)
- 4 × 25 swim on :10R (focus—hip snap and hip rhythm) descend 1-4
- IHR

WORKOUT

- TEST (LT), swim 8 × 50 on 3:00 (or 6 on 4:00, 1:00Cut) w/25s EZ drill and swim mix on :10R [fast2, slow, avgS/L]

IHR

Cool-Down

- 8-minute set, EZ 50s on :10RMax—Alt 25 SGBB weak / swim 25 (focus—side skating)
- 2 × 25 swim on :15R both @–3S/L

IHR

TOTAL YARDAGE: assuming 1:20/100 cruise pace, approximately 2,400 yards; assuming 1:40/100 cruise pace, approximately 1,900 yards; assuming 2:00/100 cruise pace, approximately 1,600 yards

COMMENTS

Although the main set doesn't look like much yardage, done properly as all-out effort 50s, this set will be stressful. Be sure to do the entire cool-down after the main set. Do more EZ swimming if you have not substantially recovered by the end of the cool-down.

9

TOTAL TIME: 40-50 minutes

TARGET HEART RATE RANGE: 75-100% of max heart rate
RPE: 7-10
WARM-UP
- 6-minute set, continuous Fins—Alt 25 BBR / 25 SGBB Rt / 25 BBR / 25 SGBB Lft
- 6-minute set, continuous—Alt 25 SFS / 25 swim (focus—surge and skate, stroke count)
- IHR

WORKOUT

- 4 × 25 swim AFAP OACI

IHR
- TEST (LT), swim 4 × 100 (or 75, 2:00Cut) on 6:00 w/50s EZ drill and swim mix on IHR [fast2, slow, avgS/L]

IHR
- 4 × 25 swim FinsOpt AFAP OACI

IHR

Cool-Down
- 8-minute set, 50s on IHR (keep HR near bottom of your GATHRR)—Alt 50 swim (focus—stroke count) / 50 DChoice

IHR

TOTAL YARDAGE: assuming 1:20/100 cruise pace, approximately 2,350 yards; assuming 1:40/100 cruise pace, approximately 1,850 yards; assuming 2:00/100 cruise pace, approximately 1,550 yards

COMMENTS

Use fast fin swimming to notice where you are working against more resistance than necessary. Have you recalculated your GATHRR lately? As you get in better aerobic shape your GATHRR will change.

LACTATE TOLERANCE#3

TOTAL TIME: 40-50 minutes

TARGET HEART RATE RANGE: 75-100% of max heart rate
RPE: 7-10
WARM-UP
10-minute set:

- 3 × 100 on IHR—Alt 25 SFS / 25 SGF / 50 swim (focus— surge and skate)
- 4 × 25 swim (focus—minimum stroke count) on :10RMax
- 50s swim (focus—hip rhythm) FinsOpt—Descending on IHR to finish 10 minutes
- IHR

WORKOUT

- TEST (LT), swim 3 × 200 (or 150, 4:00Cut) on 12:00 w/100s EZ drill and swim mix on IHR [fast2, slow, avgS/L]

IHR
Cool-Down
- 10-minute set, swim 100s on IHR—start @ CPace and swim each one 1 to 3 seconds slower than the preceding one; try to decrease stroke count throughout set

TOTAL YARDAGE: assuming 1:20/100 cruise pace, approximately 2,750 yards; assuming 1:40/100 cruise pace, approximately 2,200 yards; assuming 2:00/100 cruise pace, approximately 1,850 yards

COMMENTS

During the long rest periods between the test set swims, you should evenly divide your time with EZ swimming and your choice of drills—fins are OK here. Low-intensity aerobic activity (HRs near the bottom of your GATHRR) between high-intensity repeats is referred to as *active rest*. This is an excellent opportunity for technique-focused activities.

Red Zone

The high-intensity practices in the Orange zone introduced a variety of challenging anaerobic test sets. The longer duration (up to 60 minutes) Red zone practices use these same test sets but add more aerobic swimming, mainly at cruise pace or on cruise intervals. These are the most challenging and stressful practices, and you should only undertake them when you are feeling fresh and rested.

As in the Orange practices, there will be several places to record information and results from different swimming sets.

In the Red practices, do not use fins unless the practice notation calls for them, subject to the same exceptions expressed for the Orange zone practices.

Final Focus Point

Remember not to simply toss everything you have worked so hard for; hold onto as many efficiency skills as possible while revving the hip rotation engine faster to get more speed.

- **Easy speed:** Quite simply, this is the nirvana of swimming—going fast but doing it easily. The idea is to be as relaxed as possible as you increase speed. Start with your face. When you are trying to go fast, are you grimacing or is there a look of tranquillity upon your visage? Then work down your body. Release tension in any part on the body not actively propelling you. See how little effort you can put into each motion and still have it happen rapidly.

CRUISING

TOTAL TIME: 50-60 minutes

TARGET HEART RATE RANGE: 75-90% of max heart rate

RPE: 7-9

WARM-UP

- 6-minute set, drill and swim continuous SBFinsOpt—Alt 25 FB / 25 SGB weak / 25 swim (focus—choice)
- 6-minute set, swim 50s at CPace on :5 to :10R
- IHR

WORKOUT

- 18-minute set, swim 200s (or 150s) on CInt LOFO

IHR

- Swim 100 EZ

IHR

- 12-minute set, swim 100s (or 75s) on CInt LOFO

IHR

- Swim 100 EZ

IHR

- 6-minute set, swim 50s (or 25s) on CInt LOFO

IHR

Cool-Down

- 6-minute set, 100s on :10RMax—Alt 25 SGBB / 50 SGF / 25 swim (focus—choice)

TOTAL YARDAGE: assuming 1:20/100 cruise pace, approximately 3,700 yards; assuming 1:40/100 cruise pace, approximately 2,950 yards; assuming 2:00/100 cruise pace, approximately 2,450 yards

COMMENTS

If you would like to be able to do some CInt and CPace sets with fins, do a T-swim with fins to establish chart listing benchmarks. The EZ 100s during the main set are intended to give you short periods of active rest during this long, anaerobic threshold training set. Do not take extra rest beyond the few seconds necessary to do IHR checks.

REVIEW

2 WORKOUT

TOTAL TIME: 50-60 minutes

TARGET HEART RATE RANGE: 75-90% of max heart rate
RPE: 7-9
WARM-UP
10-minute set:

- 1 × 25 FB
- 1 × 25 BB
- 1 × 50 SGB—Alt 25 Rt / 25 Lft
- 1 × 50 SGBB—Alt 25 Rt / 25 Lft
- 1 × 50 BBR—Alt 25 roll 360s to the Rt / 25 roll 360s to the Lft
- 1 × 25 SFS

- 1 × 25 SGF
- 1 × 25 3&G
- 1 × 25 5&G
- 50s swim (focus—choice) descending on :10R to finish 10 minutes
- IHR

WORKOUT

- 25-minute set, swim choice of distance over 100 on CInt (focus—choice)

IHR

- 4 × 25 kick fast, fins in full streamline position on :10RMax

IHR

- 10-minute set, swim 100s (or 50s) on CInt (focus—stroke count)

IHR

- 4 × 25 kick fast, fins in full streamline position on :10RMax

IHR

- 5-minute set, swim 25s on CInt (focus—hip rhythm) LOFO

IHR

Cool-Down

- 6-minute set, continuous swim, starting at CPace and gradually getting slower while decreasing stroke count throughout the swim

IHR

TOTAL YARDAGE: assuming 1:20/100 cruise pace, approximately 3,500 yards; assuming 1:40/100 cruise pace, approximately 2,800 yards; assuming 2:00/100 cruise pace, approximately 2,350 yards

COMMENTS

No extra rest in the main set—go immediately from one item into the next. Same goes for the warm-up.

SWIMMING GOLF

TOTAL TIME: 50-60 minutes

TARGET HEART RATE RANGE: 75-90% of max heart rate
RPE: 7-9
WARM-UP
10-minute set:

- 200 (or 100) FinsOpt—
  Alt 25 SGBB weak / 25 SFS
- 200 (or 100) FinsOpt—
  Alt 25 SGBB good /
  25 swim (focus—choice)

- 200 (or 100) SBFinsOpt swim
  (focus—surge and skate)
- 50s swim (focus—consistent
  stroke count) descending on
  IHR to finish 10 minutes
- IHR

WORKOUT

- 6-minute set, swim @ CPace (choose
  a distance for which cruise time is 6
  minutes or more)

IHR

- 1 × 100 SGolf

IHR

- 14-minute set, swim 150s (or 100s)
  on CInt

IHR

- 1 × 100 SGolf (for lower score)

IHR

- 10-minute set, swim 75s (or 50s) on
  CInt

IHR

- 1 × 100 SGolf (for lower
  score)

IHR

- 6-minute set, swim 25s CInt—
  Alt 1@NS/L, 1@–1S/L

IHR

- 1 × 100 SGolf (for lower
  score)

IHR

Cool-Down

- 6-minute set, continuous EZ
  swim—Alt 50@NS/L, 50@–1S/
  L, 50@–2S/L

IHR

TOTAL YARDAGE: assuming 1:20/100 cruise pace, approximately
3,700 yards; assuming 1:40/100 cruise pace, approximately 2,950 yards;
assuming 2:00/100 cruise pace, approximately 2,450 yards

COMMENTS

No extra rest during the main set—this will make the swimming
golf 100s quite challenging.

4 WORKOUT

TOTAL TIME: 50-60 minutes

TARGET HEART RATE RANGE: 75-100% of max heart rate
RPE: 7-10
WARM-UP
- 12-minute continuous drill and swim—Alt 25 SFS / 75 swim (focus—25 long reach / 25 laser beam body-roll trigger / 25 stroke count)
- IHR

WORKOUT

- 9-minute set, swim 200s (or 150s) on CInt

IHR
- Swim 100 EZ

IHR
- TEST (LE), 16-minute set, swim 50s on 1:1 W/RInt :03Range [interval, fast2, slow, avgS/L] (perhaps an EZ 25 of drill between each fast 50, instead of just standing still)

IHR
- Swim 100 EZ

IHR
- 9-minute set, swim 150s (or 100s) on CInt LOFO

IHR

Cool-Down
- 6-minute set, EZ drill and swim 50s SBFins on :10R—Alt 50 DChoice / 50 swim

IHR

TOTAL YARDAGE: assuming 1:20/100 cruise pace, approximately 3,400 yards; assuming 1:40/100 cruise pace, approximately 2,750 yards; assuming 2:00/100 cruise pace, approximately 2,250 yards

COMMENTS

On the second 9-minute cruise interval set, choose a shorter distance than you did on the first one. Try not to allow your stroke count to increase from the first CInt set to the second.

LACTATE ENDURANCE #2

TOTAL TIME: 50-60 minutes

TARGET HEART RATE RANGE: 75-100% of max heart rate
RPE: 7-10
WARM-UP

- 12-minute set, swim 100s (focus—stroke count; don't let it go up) on IHR; start slow and gradually increase intensity so HR moves from bottom of GATHRR to top of GATHRR

WORKOUT

- 16-minute set, swim (choice of distance) on CInt (focus—stroke count) LOFO

IHR

- 2 × 50 EZ DChoice on :10R

IHR

- TEST (LE), 18-minute set, swim 75s on 1:1 W/RInt :03Range [interval, fast2, slow, avgS/L] (perhaps go an EZ 50 of SFS during the rest between each fast 75)

IHR
Cool-Down

- 8-minute set, 100s FinsOpt SGF on IHR, keep HR near bottom of GATHRR

TOTAL YARDAGE: assuming 1:20/100 cruise pace, approximately 3,350 yards; assuming 1:40/100 cruise pace, approximately 2,650 yards; assuming 2:00/100 cruise pace, approximately 2,200 yards

COMMENTS

Try to start the test set at a lower stroke count than your average from the last time you did this test set. Then don't let the stroke count go up.

6 W
O
R
K
O
U
T

TOTAL TIME: 50-60 minutes

TARGET HEART RATE RANGE: 75-100% of max heart rate
RPE: 7-10
WARM-UP
11-minute set:

- 2 × 50 on :10R—Alt 25 SBDChoice / 25 swim (focus—choice)
- 2 × 50 on :10R—Alt 25 DBDChoice / 25 swim (focus—choice)
- 2 × 50 on :10R—Alt 25 SIDChoice / 25 swim (focus—choice)
- 50s swim (focus—25 hip rhythm / 25 easy speed) on :10R to finish 11 minutes
- IHR

WORKOUT

- 9 × 50 SGolf on :45Rmax (focus—easy speed)

IHR

- 8-minute set, swim continuous EZ—Alt 50@NS/L, 50@−2S/L

IHR

- TEST (LE), 20-minute set, swim 100s on 1:1 W/RInt :04Range [interval, fast2, slow, avgS/L] (perhaps go an EZ 75 or 50 of SGF or SGBB during the rest between each fast 100)

IHR

Cool-Down

- 6-minute set, swim 50s on CInt (just make the interval)

IHR

TOTAL YARDAGE: assuming 1:20/100 cruise pace, approximately 3,150 yards; assuming 1:40/100 cruise pace, approximately 2,500 yards; assuming 2:00/100 cruise pace, approximately 2,100 yards

COMMENTS

Before you start this practice, look up the results of your previous SGolf sets and calculate an average score per 50 repeat. Use this as your par on the 9 × 50 SGolf set, and see if you can go through this 9-hole course, ending up under par for the whole course.

LACTATE ENDURANCE #4

TOTAL TIME: 50-60 minutes

TARGET HEART RATE RANGE: 75-100% of max heart rate
RPE: 7-10
WARM-UP
10-minute set:

- 2 × 100 (or 75 or 50) swim Fins on IHR (focus—choice)
- 2 × 100 (or 75 or 50) swim SBFins on IHR (focus—choice)
- 2 × 100 (or 75 or 50) swim (focus—choice) on IHR
- 25s swim on :5 to :10R (focus—easy speed) descending to finish 10-minute set
- IHR

WORKOUT

- TEST (LE), 24-minute set, swim 200s on 1:1 W/RInt :06Range [interval, fast2, slow, avgS/L] (perhaps alternating 25 swim (low stroke count) and 25 SGBB between fast 200s)

IHR

- 1 × 100 EZ swim—Count your total strokes for this swim

IHR

15-minute CInt set:

- Swim 4 × 100 (or 75) on CInt
- Swim 4 × 75 (or 50) on CInt
- Swim 50s (or 25s) on CInt to finish 15 minutes LOFO (focus—easy speed)

IHR

- 1 × 100 swim—How fast can you go using no more strokes than in previous EZ 100?

IHR

Cool-Down

6-minute set:

- 4 × 50 on :10R Fins—Alt 25 SGBB / 25 SIDChoice
- EZ 50s swim on :05R (focus—hand swapping) to finish 6 minutes

IHR

TOTAL YARDAGE: assuming 1:20/100 cruise pace, approximately 3,450 yards; assuming 1:40/100 cruise pace, approximately 2,800 yards; assuming 2:00/100 cruise pace, approximately 2,300 yards

COMMENTS

There is no extra rest between lines of the 15-minute cruise interval set—go immediately from one line to the next.

8

TOTAL TIME: 50-60 minutes

TARGET HEART RATE RANGE: 75-100% of max heart rate
RPE: 7-10
WARM-UP

- 4-minute set, drill and swim continuous SBFinsOpt—Alt 25 DChoice / 25 swim
- 4-minute set, swim CPace 50s on :10RMax (focus—choice)
- 4-minute set, swim 25s on :10R (focus—choice) descending
- 4-minute set, swim 50s FinsOpt on :10R (focus—choice) descending
- IHR

WORKOUT

- TEST (LT), swim 8 × 50 on 3:00 (or 6 on 4:00, 1:00Cut) w/25s EZ drill and swim mix on :10R [fast2, slow, avgS/L]

IHR
- 1 × 100 EZ swim

IHR
- 12-minute set, swim 100s @ CPace on :10R (or 50s @ CPace on :05R) LOFO; try to reduce stroke count through this set

IHR
Cool-Down
- 5-minute set, EZ 50s continuous—Alt 25 SGBB weak / swim 25 (focus—choice)
- 2 × 25 swim on :15R both @–3S/L

IHR

TOTAL YARDAGE: assuming 1:20/100 cruise pace, approximately 3,400 yards; assuming 1:40/100 cruise pace, approximately 2,700 yards; assuming 2:00/100 cruise pace, approximately 2,250 yards

COMMENTS

The test set followed by the CPace set gives an excellent opportunity to focus on efficient swimming while you are fatigued. Note that the focus for each swim is Choice. This means you select a focus that you need in your stroke. Keep shifting your focus, spending more time correcting and refining problem areas, rather than focusing on what is already working well.

LACTATE TOLERANCE#2

TOTAL TIME: 50-60 minutes

TARGET HEART RATE RANGE: 75-100% of max heart rate
RPE: 7-10
WARM-UP
- 6-minute set, continuous Fins—Alt 25 SGBB weak / 25 swim (focus—choice)
- 6-minute set, continuous—Alt 25 SGF / 25 swim (focus—stroke count; each 25 in fewer strokes than the previous 25 swim)
- IHR

WORKOUT

- 12-minute set, swim 2 × 500 (or shorter distance) @ CPace on 1:00 rest (choose a distance with CPace time at 5:30 or less)

IHR
- 4 × 25 swim FinsOpt AFAP OACI

IHR
- TEST (LT), swim 4 × 100 (or 75, 2:00Cut) on 6:00 w/50s EZ drill and swim mix on IHR [fast2, slow, avgS/L]

IHR
- 4 × 25 swim FinsOpt AFAP OACI (focus—easy speed)

IHR

Cool-Down
- 6-minute set, 50s on IHR (keep HR near bottom of your GATHRR)— Alt 50 Swim (focus—stroke count) / 50 DChoice

IHR

TOTAL YARDAGE: assuming 1:20/100 cruise pace, approximately 3,150 yards; assuming 1:40/100 cruise pace, approximately 2,500 yards; assuming 2:00/100 cruise pace, approximately 2,100 yards

COMMENTS

On the 12-minute CPace set, see how little energy you can put into swimming at your CPace. The idea is to see how low a HR you can keep during that set. Be sure to take an IHR at the beginning of the 1:00 rest as well as at the end.

10

**W
O
R
K
O
U
T**

TOTAL TIME: 50-60 minutes

TARGET HEART RATE RANGE: 75-100% of max heart rate
RPE: 7-10
WARM-UP
10-minute set:

- 3 × 100 on IHR—Alt 25 SFS / 25 SGF / 50 swim (focus—choice)
- 4 × 25 swim (focus—stroke count; each one should be fewer strokes than the previous one) on :10RMax
- 50s swim FinsOpt descending on IHR to finish 10 minutes
- IHR

WORKOUT

- 8-minute set, swim 25s @ CPace on :5 to :10R—Keep same stroke count throughout

IHR
- TEST (LT), swim 3 × 200 (or 150, 4:00Cut) on 12:00 w/100s EZ drill and swim mix on IHR [fast2, slow, avgS/L]

IHR
- 5-minute set, swim 25s @ CPace on :5 to :10R LOFO; use one fewer S/L than in 8-minute set

IHR
Cool-Down
- 6-minute set, swim 75s on IHR, start @ CPace and swim each one 1 or 2 seconds slower than the preceding one; decrease stroke count throughout set

TOTAL YARDAGE: assuming 1:20/100 cruise pace, approximately 3,150 yards; assuming 1:40/100 cruise pace, approximately 2,500 yards; assuming 2:00/100 cruise pace, approximately 2,100 yards

COMMENTS

Now that you have done each of the LE and LT test sets with no fins, you may do some of them with short-blade fins for more variety. Be sure to record these results separately from your naked test sets

PART III

TRAINING BY THE WORKOUT ZONES

Part II introduced you to a variety of practices that involve technique and conditioning activities in progressively longer or more intense sessions. Once you have familiarized yourself with the skill drills, technique concepts, and practice notation, you are ready to embark on a rest-of-your-life aquatic adventure. Part III will help you do that. In the following chapters, you'll learn how to organize the practices into a training program and chart your progress.

I encourage you to think of the practices in part II as brush strokes on a canvas. The colors you choose and how you put them together will determine what the picture looks like during the painting process.

Chapter 12 will give you a conceptual basis for putting together a seasonal training program that incorporates different training phases and appropriate amounts of rest. In addition, I offer specific examples of how many swimmers, competitive or otherwise, organize their training.

Chapter 13 offers a variety of sample three-week programs that you can use as the building blocks of an entire season. The sample programs in chapter 13 are based on three levels of interest and ability:

- **Beginning and easy.** These programs consist mainly of Green and Blue zone practices, which keep the focus on skill drills. They are designed to teach and reinforce the fundamentals of efficient freestyle swimming, while addressing the need for aerobic activity three or four practices per week. Although most of these practices are intended to keep your heart rate in the lower end of the aerobic training heart rate range, there are also a few Purple and Yellow practices, which are more intense.

- **Frequent and moderate.** Frequent swimmers go beyond the minimum aerobic exercise requirements, training more often, for longer periods, and at higher intensities. If you swim four or five times per week, you are most likely in this category. These programs allow more full-stroke swimming and lead up to the more stressful, competitive workouts. Frequent swimmers may do an occasional competition, such as an open-water swim or entering a distance event at a local Masters meet.

- **Competitive and intense.** If you find that your system requires a daily fix of chlorine fumes to feel just right, then you belong in this category. Whether you compete in meets is immaterial. A competitive swimmer is one who finds joy and motivation in testing speed and endurance, whether against the pace clock or against another chlorine animal. The workouts in these programs are designed for swimmers who want to swim fast now and faster next week. They are intense and provide a progressive challenge.

If you choose to use the programs in chapter 13, you will find they are progressive, continually testing your skill, endurance, and speed. If you decide to create your own program, I encourage you to follow the order of the practices in any color zone, at least until you have done each practice in that zone once. After that you'll be able to mix and match them.

Chapter 14 explains how to keep your motivation high by accurately tracking your swimming progress day to day, week to week, and season to season. Several handy progress charts are supplied for you to photocopy and take to the pool.

12

Setting Up Your Program

Setting up a training program is a balancing act between work and rest. The sample programs in chapter 13 typically lay out training days, alternating between less and more intense days. Too many intense days in a row or in a week will leave you stale at best and sick or injured at worst. Overtraining, for any athlete, has potentially far worse consequences than undertraining.

Take a Day Off

Regardless of your ability level, conditioning level, or interest level, you should take at least one day off completely from swimming each week. This will help keep both your body and your mind fresher when you are in the pool. Pursuing other physical activities on your day off is fine as long as you keep the stress-level low. Consider this another form of active rest.

Elements of a Swim Training Program

Most lap swimmers get into a habit of doing long swims at the same moderate pace, with little or no technique in their workout. They do this every time they go to the pool. That is a sure-fire plan for becoming better conditioned to swim slowly with the same ugly stroke you've always used.

If you want to become a better and faster swimmer, you have to use a different strategy. There are four types of training that form the building blocks of this strategy. These building blocks combine a progression of conditioning phases (general, specific, competitive, and taper), with a progression of skill-acquisition phases (learning, practicing, and monitoring). How you stack those building blocks determines the outcome of your efforts.

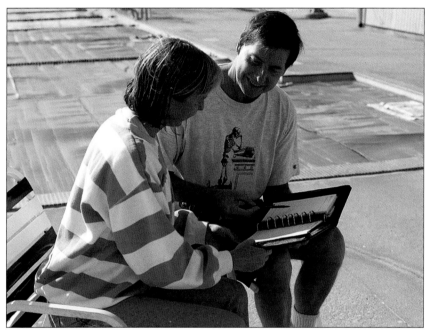

Planning ahead allows you to make the most effective use of your training time.

Technique Acquisition and Endurance

Basic endurance for swimming is the ability to go through the motions of efficient swimming at submaximal paces for extended periods. Any training season must start at this level to successfully negotiate more demanding training regimens. Even elite swimmers spend the first several months of each training season learning new swimming skills and increasing sensitivity to skill nuances. Learning new skills while laying down a base of aerobic conditioning with skill drills and focused, low-intensity swimming should constitute a sizable portion of your training.

Technique Refinement and Specific Endurance Phase

Once you establish basic endurance, it is time to increase the intensity of the aerobic training. This involves introducing and progressively increasing anaerobic threshold training, using cruise pace and cruise interval training. For swimmers with no competitive or risk-taking bent, this may be as far as they ever want to venture into swim conditioning. Still, intermixed with this higher conditioning are large quantities of skill drills and technique-focused swimming sets. With the intention of refining skills acquired in the basic endurance phase, use "practice makes permanent" as the technique theme for this training phase.

Technique Maintenance and Competition Phase

If you are going to compete or test your body's limits, then your season will include this phase. Lactate endurance and lactate tolerance work will be the conditioning focus, but there is still enough endurance work to avoid losing aerobic conditioning. There should also be an anaerobic alactic component (pure speed, short sprints, lots of rest) during this phase of training. If you compete, schedule most of your competitions during this training period, because they will serve as a portion of your high-intensity training. During this phase of training, your technique focus shifts toward maintaining the skills you have acquired and refined during earlier training. This involves doing skill drill work but includes more full-stroke swimming using real-time feedback tools. Monitoring your application and execution of efficient swimming skills is the technique theme for this phase of training.

Tapering

If you are a competitor, you likely have some specific season-culminating competition that you are training toward. A training season is planned to allow one's best performance during this culminating activity. A training taper is a period of reduced training stress, during which the body supercompensates in a variety of physiological systems. During taper, a swimmer may cut total training volume (yardage and duration) to as little as one-third of pretaper volume. The key is to maintain the same relative intensity work as in pretaper practices—just do less of it. Competitive swimmers routinely report dramatic improvements in their tapered performances over untapered performances.

Taking Time Off

Regardless of your reasons for swimming, an occasional break from your training program—from a week up to a month—is necessary to maintain freshness and enthusiasm. When you return to the pool, you will have a renewed outlook on your conditioning and technique-acquisition efforts.

Exercise and Adaptation

It is a common misconception that the work you do in a practice makes you a better conditioned swimmer. In fact, it is what you do between work sessions—during your recovery periods—that makes you a better conditioned swimmer.

Under normal conditions, the human body automatically makes positive adaptations in response to physical demands. Your body seeks a state in which the physical activities you regularly engage in are not a great hardship. If you are a furniture mover, your body will add muscle mass to help you lift heavy objects. If you run five miles every day, your body will increase the aerobic capacity of the muscles in your legs and improve your cardiovascular system. Exercise sends signals to your brain and body that can trigger a variety of physiological adaptations, meaning greater strength, more explosiveness, more endurance, and so on.

The operative phrase in the previous paragraph is "under normal conditions," which include proper nutrition, proper hydration, adequate amounts of high-quality sleep, minimal or zero amounts of cultural pollutants (alcohol, nicotine, crack, potato chips) in the bloodstream, freedom from disease, and relatively low psychological stress levels.

Lack of sleep is probably the most common and most destructive deviation from ideal adaptation conditions. If you are getting little sleep, you'd probably be better off to take the two or three hours you now devote to the workout process (traveling, training, and traveling again) and invest it in a good solid nap. Better yet, get to bed earlier.

Constantly infringing on the ideal adaptation conditions will mean you are spotting your competition a huge advantage. If you work out regularly and passionately, yet insist on living the rest of your life like John Belushi, you can expect to eat serious wake.

Your Yearly Training Plan

Here is a periodized training schedule for a typical Masters training season, focused at a peak performance at Short-Course (25-yard pool) Nationals in mid-May.

Planning a season starts with the end in mind. We'll plan backward from that mid-May date. Because Long-Course (50-meter pool) Nationals usually take place in mid-August and swimmers often take a month off after the big meet, the earliest we might start a short-course training season would be in mid-September—a total of 35 weeks.

- **Taper period.** Depending on the intensity and duration of the training season, taper should last anywhere from two to four weeks. We'll take a middle ground of three weeks from late April to mid-May.

Personal experience over a few seasons will give you a better idea of how long your taper should be.

- **Competition period.** Depending on the duration of your training season, your competition training period could be from 6 to 12 weeks. This is the optimum duration range for concentrated, high-intensity training. Ideally, after deducting the taper period we have roughly 32 weeks left in our season. We want each endurance training phase to be longer than our competition phase, so we'll block out the 9 weeks from mid-February until late April, less than one-third of the remaining season, for our competition training.

- **Specific endurance.** With 23 weeks remaining for endurance training, we want to spend half in each endurance phase. So, for our specific endurance period, we'll block out 12 weeks—December through mid-February—knowing that we'll probably lose a week of training around the holidays.

- **Basic endurance.** This leaves the 11 weeks from mid-September through the end of November for our basic endurance period.

Specific Training Programs

Several training programs that you can use to prepare for the Short-Course Nationals or Long-Course Nationals are presented here. Keep in mind that these programs are not set in stone. Each individual has specific preparatory needs.

TRAINING PROGRAMS FOR COMPETITION PREPARATION

A 35-week Short-Course Nationals season looks like this:

Basic endurance	11 weeks (mid-September through the end of November)
Specific endurance	12 weeks (December until mid-February)
Competition period	9 weeks (mid-February to late April)
Taper	3 weeks (late April to mid-May)
Short-Course Nationals	
Break	2 weeks (until early June)

If you then wanted to go to Long-Course Nationals in mid-August, you would have a laughably short season of 11 weeks to work with. You might arrange it as follows:

Cut break short	1 week—this gives you 12 weeks to work with
Basic endurance	3 weeks (late May to mid-June)
Specific endurance	4 weeks (mid-June to early July)
Competition period	3 weeks (early July to very late July)
Taper	2 weeks (very late July to mid-August)
Long-Course Nationals	
Break	4 weeks (until mid-September)

By no means is this an ideal scenario for a training season, but it illustrates how you execute the principles for building a season at the extreme short end of the spectrum.

Some swimmers and coaches prefer to plan three seasons in a year rather than two. A **three-season** yearly cycle might look like this.

Season 1
15 weeks from early September culminating in a selected meet in late December:

Basic endurance	4 weeks (early September until early October)
Specific endurance	5 weeks (early October until early November)
Competition period	4 weeks (early November until early December)
Taper	2 weeks (early December until late December)
Selected Meet	
1 or 2 weeks break	

Season 2
20 weeks from January 1st culminating in Short-Course Nationals in mid-May:

Basic endurance	6 weeks (January through mid-February)
Specific endurance	6 weeks (mid-February until late March)
Competition period	5 weeks (late March until late April)
Taper	3 weeks (late April to mid-May)
Short-Course Nationals	
1 or 2 weeks break	

Season 3
11 or 12 weeks long-course training season as described earlier with three- to four-week break.

13

Sample Swimming Programs

Most adults who swim will say that they do it first and foremost for fitness. After that, there are many reasons that humans venture into the water. Whether you desire the rudiments of aerobic fitness, want to increase the effectiveness of your swimming, or are motivated to train for the National Championships, read on. If chlorine and a black line are staples of your water experience, you will find a set of programs here that can help you in your quest.

Beginning and Easy Swimming Programs (Lap and Fitness Swimming)

As a beginning swimmer, you probably head to the pool regularly for relaxation and enjoyment or as part of your overall aerobic fitness plan. The beginning and easy programs give you variety and learning activities while enhancing your aerobic fitness.

Improving Technique

These two programs present the complete set of Green and Blue practices in a logical progression, slowly introducing new skill drills and gradually increasing yardage and complexity. If you are new to this system, scored average or below average on your T-15 swim, scored low on the fitness evaluation, are a beginning swimmer, or if any of the skill drills or training concepts are foreign to you, I strongly encourage you to start with these programs. The last day of each program calls for you to repeat an easier practice, followed by another T-15 swim (recording your results).

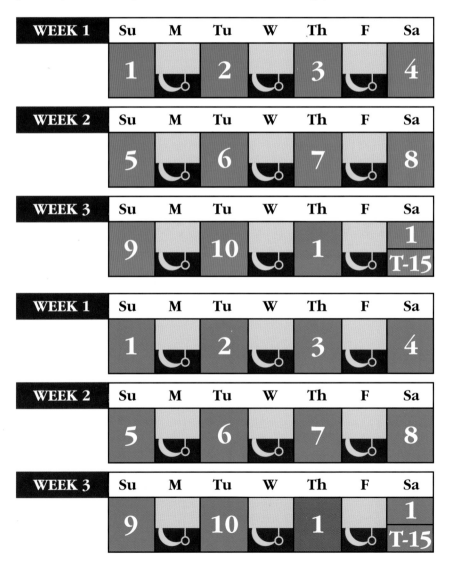

If your fitness level is above average but you still need to acquaint yourself with the skill drills in a logical learning order, consider accelerating the progression by taking fewer days off or by doing two practices on some days. In either case, I recommend you do the practices in the order indicated. If your schedule allows time enough for only three practices per week, lengthen these programs to four weeks, but follow the order indicated.

Building Endurance

It's time to start building your endurance after you have gone through the Green and Blue practices at least once and are familiar with the drills and focus points. These two programs give you flexibility while gradually introducing more challenging practices. Note that 1-5 in a green box, for example, means to select one practice from Green 1 through Green 5.

WEEK 1	Su	M	Tu	W	Th	F	Sa
	1-4		1		5-7		2

WEEK 2	Su	M	Tu	W	Th	F	Sa
	8-10		3		1-4		4

WEEK 3	Su	M	Tu	W	Th	F	Sa
	5-7		5		8-10		T-15 1

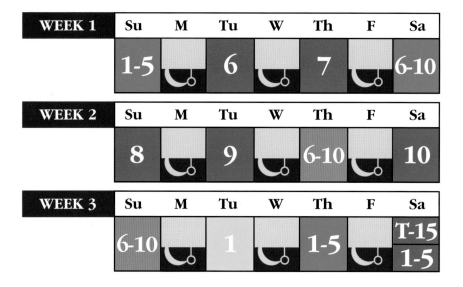

WEEK 1	Su	M	Tu	W	Th	F	Sa
	1-5		6		7		6-10

WEEK 2	Su	M	Tu	W	Th	F	Sa
	8		9		6-10		10

WEEK 3	Su	M	Tu	W	Th	F	Sa
	6-10		1		1-5		T-15 1-5

Frequent Swimming Programs (Precompetitive)

Swimmers who have been regular in their workout habits soon want to increase their frequency and intensity—often with an eye toward competing in the future. The frequent, precompetitive workouts increase training volume, frequency, and intensity while laying the groundwork for more intense training for competition.

Improving Technique

In these programs the frequency goes up to five practices per week, including more Purple and Yellow practices with more yardage and intensity. These are interspersed with lower intensity, fundamental skill practices from the Green and Blue zones. The first two Saturdays of each program are longer days, using an easy Green practice as a warm-up for a more intense Purple or Yellow practice. As before, the final Saturday of each program calls for a T-15 swim.

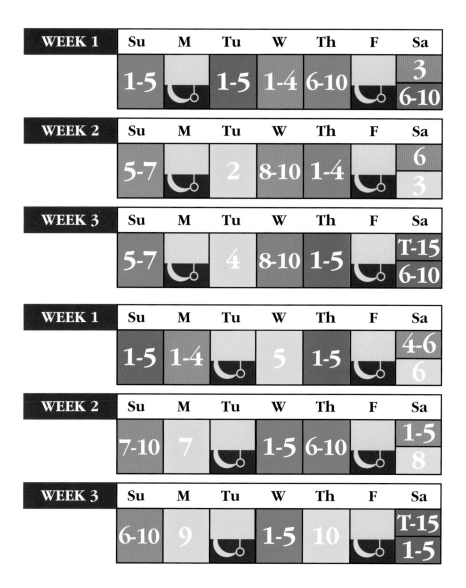

WEEK 1	Su	M	Tu	W	Th	F	Sa
	1-5		1-5	1-4	6-10		3 / 6-10

WEEK 2	Su	M	Tu	W	Th	F	Sa
	5-7		2	8-10	1-4		6 / 3

WEEK 3	Su	M	Tu	W	Th	F	Sa
	5-7		4	8-10	1-5		T-15 / 6-10

WEEK 1	Su	M	Tu	W	Th	F	Sa
	1-5	1-4		5	1-5		4-6 / 6

WEEK 2	Su	M	Tu	W	Th	F	Sa
	7-10	7		1-5	6-10		1-5 / 8

WEEK 3	Su	M	Tu	W	Th	F	Sa
	6-10	9		1-5	10		T-15 / 1-5

Building Endurance

These programs call for five practices per week, adding one or two Orange practices per week to the mix of Purple, Yellow, Green, and Blue practices. Saturdays continue to be longer days. There will be longer anaerobic threshold sets and some lactate endurance sets. Many Orange practices involve test sets other than the T-swims you have been doing. These involve more record keeping to track your progress. Note the final

Saturday of the second program calls for a T-20 swim instead of a T-15 swim.

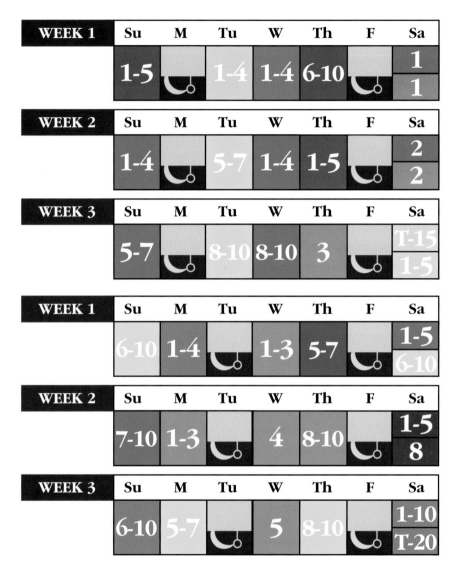

Building Speed

These programs will build your speed with more lactate endurance work and maximize and test your speed with lactate tolerance work. Note that these practice days (Red 4-10 and Orange 4-10) are followed by either a rest day or a low- or moderate-intensity Green, Blue, or Purple day.

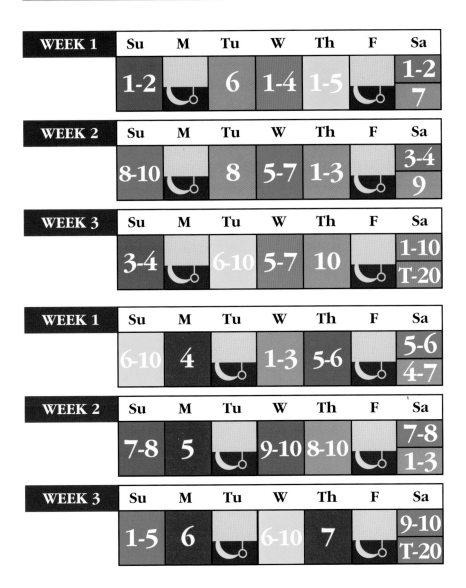

WEEK 1	Su	M	Tu	W	Th	F	Sa
	1-2		6	1-4	1-5		1-2 / 7

WEEK 2	Su	M	Tu	W	Th	F	Sa
	8-10		8	5-7	1-3		3-4 / 9

WEEK 3	Su	M	Tu	W	Th	F	Sa
	3-4		6-10	5-7	10		1-10 / T-20

WEEK 1	Su	M	Tu	W	Th	F	Sa
	6-10	4		1-3	5-6		5-6 / 4-7

WEEK 2	Su	M	Tu	W	Th	F	Sa
	7-8	5		9-10	8-10		7-8 / 1-3

WEEK 3	Su	M	Tu	W	Th	F	Sa
	1-5	6		6-10	7		9-10 / T-20

Intense Swimming Programs (Competitive)

Either you already compete, want to compete in the near future, or just want to know what your body is capable of. In any case, a more intense program is what you are looking for. These programs assume that swimming is your primary physical activity and that you are willing to commit to more training time each week.

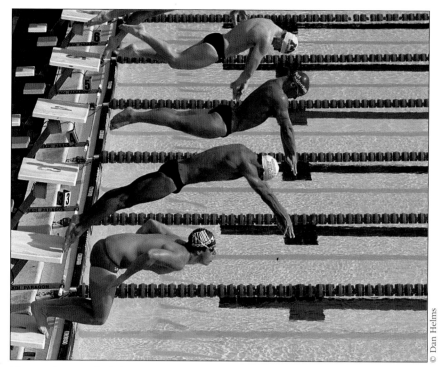

© Dan Helms

Many swimmers find that competing in their chosen sport provides extra incentive to stay with their training regimen.

Improving Technique

In these programs the frequency goes up to six practices per week, including more Orange and Red practices with more yardage and intensity. These are interspersed with lower intensity fundamental skills and conditioning workouts from the Green through Yellow zones. If your schedule does not permit six practices per week, then stretch these programs to four weeks of five practices, but keep the same order. The T-swims have now been lengthened to T-30.

WEEK 1	Su	M	Tu	W	Th	F	Sa
	1-3		1-3	1-3	4-6	4-6	5-10 / 1-5

WEEK 2	Su	M	Tu	W	Th	F	Sa
	1-3		7-10	7-10	4-5	5-10	1-3 / 6-7

WEEK 3	Su	M	Tu	W	Th	F	Sa
	1-3		5-10	5-10	5-10	5-10	1-5 / T-30

WEEK 1	Su	M	Tu	W	Th	F	Sa
	1-3	4-6	4-5		5-6	7-10	5-6 / 1-3

WEEK 2	Su	M	Tu	W	Th	F	Sa
	7-8	6-7	8-10		6-7	1-3	7-8 / 1-3

WEEK 3	Su	M	Tu	W	Th	F	Sa
	1-5	1-3	1-3		5-10	4-6	6-10 / T-30

Building Endurance

As before, we add more anaerobic threshold activities and some lactate endurance work. With only one day off each week, it becomes important to watch for signs of overtraining. If you find you are not recovering from one high-intensity workout to the next, you might stretch these programs over four weeks, adding another day of rest each week.

WEEK 1	Su	M	Tu	W	Th	F	Sa
	1-4		1-3	1-4	6-10	5-7	1-5 / 1-3

WEEK 2	Su	M	Tu	W	Th	F	Sa
	4-5		6-7	1-4	1-5	8-10	6-10 / 1-3

WEEK 3	Su	M	Tu	W	Th	F	Sa
	6-10		4-7	8-10	1-3	1-10	1-10 / T-30

WEEK 1	Su	M	Tu	W	Th	F	Sa
	6-10	4-7	1-4	5-7		1-3	1-5 / 1-3

WEEK 2	Su	M	Tu	W	Th	F	Sa
	7-10	1-3	1-4	4-7		8-10	6-10 / 1-3

WEEK 3	Su	M	Tu	W	Th	F	Sa
	6-10	8-10	5-7	1-3		5-7	1-10 / T-30

Building Speed

More lactate endurance and lactate tolerance make these programs challenging and stressful. Do not use these programs for more than 9 to 12 weeks at a time without returning to less stressful programs for a few weeks.

WEEK 1	Su	M	Tu	W	Th	F	Sa
	6-10	4-7		1-3	6	1-5	5-6 / 4-7

WEEK 2	Su	M	Tu	W	Th	F	Sa
	7-8	7		6-7	8	6-10	7-8 / 4-7

WEEK 3	Su	M	Tu	W	Th	F	Sa
	1-5	9		1-10	10	1-10	5-10 / T-30

WEEK 1	Su	M	Tu	W	Th	F	Sa
	6-10	4-7	1-10		8-10	5-6	5-6 / 1-3

WEEK 2	Su	M	Tu	W	Th	F	Sa
	1-5	4-7	6-10		8-10	1-10	7-8 / 4-7

WEEK 3	Su	M	Tu	W	Th	F	Sa
	1-5	7-10	7-10		1-3	1-10	9-10 / T-30

14

Charting
Your Progress

Most people who begin an exercise program drop out within six months. If you did not intend to be in the minority in this respect, you wouldn't have purchased this book. Yet we all know that intentions are not enough. Many things can get between you and your fitness goals—time, logistics, job, family, motivation, and so on. Although this book can't help you with the first four items on that list, it can help with the fifth. One primary reason that people drop out of an exercise program is lack of motivation. When you first begin a new program there is usually a period of two or three months in which the stimulation of new surroundings, new people, and new experiences keeps you excited about the activity. However, as the workout routine gets to be the same-old-same-old, keeping motivated gets harder.

If you have a constant supply of accurate feedback about the results of your efforts, you will find that staying motivated is easy. The more positive feedback you can get, the more excited you will be about going back to the pool for your next swim session.

That is where charting your progress comes in. Frequently throughout the programs and practices, you will have the opportunity to test various aspects of your swimming. Rather than trusting the results to memory, I strongly encourage you to start from day one recording your results and keeping these records in an organized and logical fashion.

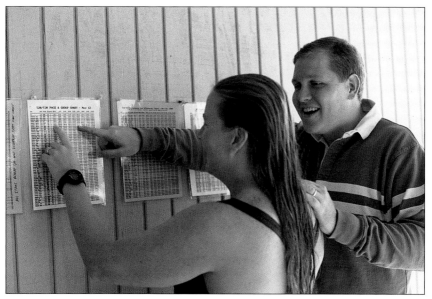

Charting and tracking your swimming progress provides a powerful feedback mechanism that can keep you motivated.

Your efforts in this regard will pay off handsomely, both short term and over the long haul. On a daily or weekly basis, you will see improvements in your results. Where you don't see improvements, you will be aware of skills or conditioning that need extra attention. As months and seasons pass, you will see a personalized, progressive pattern of increased training intensity, because you will do much of your swimming at speeds derived directly from the results of your test swims. This type of specific, personalized feedback will greatly improve the odds that (1) you stick with it and (2) you get the results you are looking for.

Progress Charts

At the end of this section are several charts for recording the results of the test sets and swims used throughout this book. Make copies of these charts as you need them for recording results over an extended time. With each chart you may want to make several copies to use with different set variations and distances. A loose-leaf binder (preferably with a built-in calculator) will help keep an organized eye on your swimming progress.

T-Swim Test Performance Chart

This is the first chart you'll become acquainted with. Initially, you'll record your T-15 swim results from the swimming fitness test in chapter 3. After that, you'll record the results of subsequent T-15 swims. Once you move up to T-20 swims, start a new chart and, likewise, when you move to T-30s. You'll need to look up your cruise pace per 100 from the appropriate T-swim chart. Progress is indicated by the following:

1. Faster cruise pace per 100

2. Same cruise pace but lower IHR

3. Same cruise pace but lower average stroke count

4. Same cruise pace but lower perceived exertion

As you move from T-15s to T-20s to T-30s, do not be alarmed if your cruise pace suffers right after making the switch. The longer T-swims are, the more accurate estimates of true cruise pace will be, assuming you give them your best effort.

Swimming Golf Performance Chart

In chapter 3 you were introduced to swimming golf. Throughout the practices there are numerous opportunities to do SGolf swims. In addition, any time you feel like testing your level of technical ability, try a few SGolf repeats. Keep separate charts for SGolf you do over different distances. Improvements are indicated by the following:

1. Lower SGolf score

2. Same SGolf score with a lower IHR

3. Same SGolf score with lower perceived exertion

Compute your swimming golf score by adding the total number of strokes to the total number of seconds required to complete a distance. You'll note that there is a column for advanced SGolf score. This is simply your regular SGolf score plus your IHR. Comparing advanced SGolf scores gives a more accurate reading of the changes in the efficiency of your swimming.

Lactate Endurance Test Set Performance Chart

As you begin doing Orange and Red workouts you'll start using this chart. You'll need to keep four of these charts—one for each of the four LE sets that appear in the Orange and Red practices. These charts are more complex but give you a wealth of progress feedback. You will need to record the calculated average swim time (add the fastest, next fastest, and slowest swim times and divide by three) as well as the calculated range of times (subtract the fastest swim time from the slowest swim time). You may realize improvements in several ways:

1. Getting a faster calculated average
2. Keeping the same average but having a smaller range
3. Having a lower average stroke count without sacrificing speed
4. Moving up to a faster interval

As your swimming improves, you will need to move to faster intervals on LE sets. The idea for LE sets is to keep a 1:1 work-to-rest ratio for the distance you are swimming. Let's say you have been swimming 100s on a 2:30 interval, and over a time have decreased your average time from 1:15s to 1:13s. Until now you have been swimming on the correct interval. Let's say that on your next couple performances you average 1:12s or 1:11s. Assuming you are keeping all your swims within the specified range, it is probably time to drop your interval to 2:25 as this would now be closer to 1:1 work-to-rest ratio.

Lactate Tolerance Test Set Performance Chart

The most intense of our test sets appear in Orange and Red workouts. There are three LE test sets for which you'll keep charts. As with the LE charts, you will need to calculate average swim times and ranges, in the same manner as before, and record them. There are three specific progress feedback points:

1. Faster calculated average swim time
2. Same average swim time but a smaller range
3. Lower average stroke count without sacrificing speed

T-Swim Test Performance Chart

Set (circle one)   T-15   T-20   T30

Date	Distance swum	Finish time	Cruise pace per 100 (look up)	Average strokes per length	IHR

Swimming Golf (SGolf) Performance Chart

Distance (circle one)   50   100   150   200

Date	Finish time	Total seconds	Total strokes	SGolf score	IHR	Advanced SGolf score

Lactate Endurance (LE) Test Set Performance Chart

Repeat distance (circle one)

16 min of 50s	18 min of 75s	20 min of 100s	24 min of 200s
:02 range	:03 range	:04 range	:06 range

Date	Repeat interval	Fastest swim	Next fastest swim	Slowest swim	Calculated average swim time	Calculated range	Average strokes per length

Calculated average swim time = (fastest + next fastest + slowest)/3
Calculated range = slowest − fastest

Lactate Tolerance (LT) Test Set Performance Chart

Set (circle one)

6 × 50	8 × 50	4 × 75	4 × 100	3 × 150	3 × 200
on 3:00	on 4:00	on 6:00	on 6:00	on 12:00	on 12:00

Date	Fastest swim	Next fastest swim	Slowest swim	Calculated average swim time	Calculated range	Average strokes per length

Calculated average swim time = (fastest + next fastest + slowest)/3
Calculated range = slowest − fastest

Testing Charts

T-15 Cruise Pace per 100 Chart

Dist.	15:00	15:10	15:20	15:30	15:40	15:50	16:00	16:10	16:20	16:30
500	3:00	3:02	3:04	3:06	3:08	3:10	3:12	3:14	3:16	3:18
550	2:43	2:45	2:47	2:49	2:50	2:52	2:54	2:56	2:58	3:00
600	2:30	2:31	2:33	2:35	2:36	2:38	2:40	2:41	2:43	2:45
650	2:18	2:20	2:21	2:23	2:24	2:26	2:27	2:29	2:30	2:32
700	2:08	2:10	2:11	2:12	2:14	2:15	2:17	2:18	2:20	2:21
750	2:00.0	2:01	2:02	2:04	2:05	2:06	2:08	2:09	2:10	2:12
800	1:52.5	1:53.7	1:55.0	1:56.2	1:57.5	1:58.7	2:00.0	2:01	2:02	2:03
850	1:45.8	1:47.0	1:48.2	1:49.4	1:50.5	1:51.7	1:52.9	1:54.1	1:55.2	1:56.4
900	1:40.0	1:41.1	1:42.2	1:43.3	1:44.4	1:45.5	1:46.6	1:47.7	1:48.8	1:50.0
950	1:34.7	1:35.7	1:36.8	1:37.8	1:38.9	1:40.0	1:41.0	1:42.1	1:43.1	1:44.2
1000	1:30.0	1:31.0	1:32.0	1:33.0	1:34.0	1:35.0	1:36.0	1:37.0	1:38.0	1:39.0
1050	1:25.7	1:26.6	1:27.6	1:28.5	1:29.5	1:30.4	1:31.4	1:32.3	1:33.3	1:34.2
1100	1:21.8	1:22.7	1:23.6	1:24.5	1:25.4	1:26.3	1:27.2	1:28.1	1:29.0	1:30.0
1150	1:18.2	1:19.1	1:20.0	1:20.8	1:21.7	1:22.6	1:23.4	1:24.3	1:25.2	1:26.0
1200	1:15.0	1:15.8	1:16.6	1:17.5	1:18.3	1:19.1	1:20.0	1:20.8	1:21.6	1:22.5
1250	1:12.0	1:12.8	1:13.6	1:14.4	1:15.2	1:16.0	1:16.8	1:17.6	1:18.4	1:19.2
1300	1:09.2	1:10.0	1:10.7	1:11.5	1:12.3	1:13.0	1:13.8	1:14.6	1:15.3	1:16.1
1350	1:06.6	1:07.4	1:08.1	1:08.8	1:09.6	1:10.3	1:11.1	1:11.8	1:12.5	1:13.3
1400	1:04.2	1:05.0	1:05.7	1:06.4	1:07.1	1:07.8	1:08.5	1:09.2	1:10.0	1:10.7
1450	1:02.0	1:02.7	1:03.4	1:04.1	1:04.8	1:05.5	1:06.2	1:06.8	1:07.5	1:08.2
1500	1:00.0	1:00.6	1:01.3	1:02.0	1:02.6	1:03.3	1:04.0	1:04.6	1:05.3	1:06.0

T-20 Cruise Pace per 100 Chart

Dist.	20:00	20:10	20:20	20:30	20:40	20:50	21:00	21:10	21:20	21:30
700	2:51	2:52	2:54	2:55	2:57	2:58	3:00	3:01	3:02	3:04
750	2:40	2:41	2:42	2:44	2:45	2:46	2:48	2:49	2:50	2:52
800	2:30	2:31	2:32	2:33	2:35	2:36	2:37	2:38	2:40	2:41
850	2:21	2:22	2:23	2:24	2:25	2:27	2:28	2:29	2:30	2:31
900	2:13	2:14	2:15	2:16	2:17	2:18	2:20	2:21	2:22	2:23
950	2:06	2:07	2:08	2:09	2:10	2:11	2:12	2:13	2:14	2:15
1000	2:00.0	2:01	2:02	2:03	2:04	2:05	2:06	2:07	2:08	2:09
1050	1:54.2	1:55.2	1:56.1	1:57.1	1:58.0	1:59.0	2:00.0	2:00	2:01	2:02
1100	1:49.0	1:50.0	1:50.9	1:51.8	1:52.7	1:53.6	1:54.5	1:55.4	1:56.3	1:57.2
1150	1:44.3	1:45.2	1:46.0	1:46.9	1:47.8	1:48.6	1:49.5	1:50.4	1:51.3	1:52.1
1200	1:40.0	1:40.8	1:41.6	1:42.5	1:43.3	1:44.1	1:45.0	1:45.8	1:46.6	1:47.5
1250	1:36.0	1:36.8	1:37.6	1:38.4	1:39.2	1:40.0	1:40.8	1:41.6	1:42.4	1:43.2
1300	1:32.3	1:33.0	1:33.8	1:34.6	1:35.3	1:36.1	1:36.9	1:37.6	1:38.4	1:39.2
1350	1:28.8	1:29.6	1:30.3	1:31.1	1:31.8	1:32.5	1:33.3	1:34.0	1:34.8	1:35.5
1400	1:25.7	1:26.4	1:27.1	1:27.8	1:28.5	1:29.2	1:30.0	1:30.7	1:31.4	1:32.1
1450	1:22.7	1:23.4	1:24.1	1:24.8	1:25.5	1:26.2	1:26.8	1:27.5	1:28.2	1:28.9
1500	1:20.0	1:20.6	1:21.3	1:22.0	1:22.6	1:23.3	1:24.0	1:24.6	1:25.3	1:26.0
1550	1:17.4	1:18.0	1:18.7	1:19.3	1:20.0	1:20.6	1:21.2	1:21.9	1:22.5	1:23.2
1600	1:15.0	1:15.6	1:16.2	1:16.8	1:17.5	1:18.1	1:18.7	1:19.3	1:20.0	1:20.6
1650	1:12.7	1:13.3	1:13.9	1:14.5	1:15.1	1:15.7	1:16.3	1:16.9	1:17.5	1:18.1
1700	1:10.5	1:11.1	1:11.7	1:12.3	1:12.9	1:13.5	1:14.1	1:14.7	1:15.2	1:15.8
1750	1:08.5	1:09.1	1:09.7	1:10.2	1:10.8	1:11.4	1:12.0	1:12.5	1:13.1	1:13.7
1800	1:06.6	1:07.2	1:07.7	1:08.3	1:08.8	1:09.4	1:10.0	1:10.5	1:11.1	1:11.6
1850	1:04.8	1:05.4	1:05.9	1:06.4	1:07.0	1:07.5	1:08.1	1:08.6	1:09.1	1:09.7
1900	1:03.1	1:03.6	1:04.2	1:04.7	1:05.2	1:05.7	1:06.3	1:06.8	1:07.3	1:07.8
1950	1:01.5	1:02.0	1:02.5	1:03.0	1:03.5	1:04.1	1:04.6	1:05.1	1:05.6	1:06.1
2000	1:00.0	1:00.5	1:01.0	1:01.5	1:02.0	1:02.5	1:03.0	1:03.5	1:04.0	1:04.5

T-30 Cruise Pace per 100 Chart

Dist.	30:00	30:10	30:20	30:30	30:40	30:50	31:00	31:10	31:20	31:30
1000	3:00	3:01	3:02	3:03	3:04	3:05	3:06	3:07	3:08	3:09
1050	2:51	2:52	2:53	2:54	2:55	2:56	2:57	2:58	2:59	3:00
1100	2:43	2:44	2:45	2:46	2:47	2:48	2:49	2:50	2:50	2:51
1150	2:36	2:37	2:38	2:39	2:40	2:40	2:41	2:42	2:43	2:44
1200	2:30	2:30	2:31	2:32	2:33	2:34	2:35	2:35	2:36	2:37
1250	2:24	2:24	2:25	2:26	2:27	2:28	2:28	2:29	2:30	2:31
1300	2:18	2:19	2:20	2:20	2:21	2:22	2:23	2:23	2:24	2:25
1350	2:13	2:14	2:14	2:15	2:16	2:17	2:17	2:18	2:19	2:20
1400	2:08	2:09	2:10	2:10	2:11	2:12	2:12	2:13	2:14	2:15
1450	2:04	2:04	2:05	2:06	2:06	2:07	2:08	2:08	2:09	2:10
1500	2:00.0	2:00	2:01	2:02	2:02	2:03	2:04	2:04	2:05	2:06
1550	1:56.1	1:56.7	1:57.4	1:58.0	1:58.7	1:59.3	2:00.0	2:00	2:01	2:01
1600	1:52.5	1:53.1	1:53.7	1:54.3	1:55.0	1:55.6	1:56.2	1:56.8	1:57.5	1:58.1
1650	1:49.0	1:49.6	1:50.3	1:50.9	1:51.5	1:52.1	1:52.7	1:53.3	1:53.9	1:54.5
1700	1:45.8	1:46.4	1:47.0	1:47.6	1:48.2	1:48.8	1:49.4	1:50.0	1:50.5	1:51.1
1750	1:42.8	1:43.4	1:44.0	1:44.5	1:45.1	1:45.7	1:46.2	1:46.8	1:47.4	1:48.0
1800	1:40.0	1:40.5	1:41.1	1:41.6	1:42.2	1:42.7	1:43.3	1:43.8	1:44.4	1:45.0
1850	1:37.2	1:37.8	1:38.3	1:38.9	1:39.4	1:40.0	1:40.5	1:41.0	1:41.6	1:42.1
1900	1:34.7	1:35.2	1:35.7	1:36.3	1:36.8	1:37.3	1:37.8	1:38.4	1:38.9	1:39.4
1950	1:32.3	1:32.8	1:33.3	1:33.8	1:34.3	1:34.8	1:35.3	1:35.8	1:36.4	1:36.9
2000	1:30.0	1:30.5	1:31.0	1:31.5	1:32.0	1:32.5	1:33.0	1:33.5	1:34.0	1:34.5
2050	1:27.8	1:28.2	1:28.7	1:29.2	1:29.7	1:30.2	1:30.7	1:31.2	1:31.7	1:32.1
2100	1:25.7	1:26.1	1:26.6	1:27.1	1:27.6	1:28.0	1:28.5	1:29.0	1:29.5	1:30.0
2150	1:23.7	1:24.1	1:24.6	1:25.1	1:25.5	1:26.0	1:26.5	1:26.9	1:27.4	1:27.9

2200	1:21.8	1:22.2	1:22.7	1:23.1	1:23.6	1:24.0	1:24.5	1:25.0	1:25.4	1:25.9
2250	1:20.0	1:20.4	1:20.8	1:21.3	1:21.7	1:22.2	1:22.6	1:23.1	1:23.5	1:24.0
2300	1:18.2	1:18.6	1:19.1	1:19.5	1:20.0	1:20.4	1:20.8	1:21.3	1:21.7	1:22.1
2350	1:16.5	1:17.0	1:17.4	1:17.8	1:18.2	1:18.7	1:19.1	1:19.5	1:20.0	1:20.4
2400	1:15.0	1:15.4	1:15.8	1:16.2	1:16.6	1:17.0	1:17.5	1:17.9	1:18.3	1:18.7
2450	1:13.4	1:13.8	1:14.2	1:14.6	1:15.1	1:15.5	1:15.9	1:16.3	1:16.7	1:17.1
2500	1:12.0	1:12.4	1:12.8	1:13.2	1:13.6	1:14.0	1:14.4	1:14.8	1:15.2	1:15.6
2550	1:10.5	1:10.9	1:11.3	1:11.7	1:12.1	1:12.5	1:12.9	1:13.3	1:13.7	1:14.1
2600	1:09.2	1:09.6	1:10.0	1:10.3	1:10.7	1:11.1	1:11.5	1:11.9	1:12.3	1:12.6
2650	1:07.9	1:08.3	1:08.6	1:09.0	1:09.4	1:09.8	1:10.1	1:10.5	1:10.9	1:11.3
2700	1:06.6	1:07.0	1:07.4	1:07.7	1:08.1	1:08.5	1:08.8	1:09.2	1:09.6	1:10.0
2750	1:05.4	1:05.8	1:06.1	1:06.5	1:06.9	1:07.2	1:07.6	1:08.0	1:08.3	1:08.7
2800	1:04.2	1:04.6	1:05.0	1:05.3	1:05.7	1:06.0	1:06.4	1:06.7	1:07.1	1:07.5
2850	1:03.1	1:03.5	1:03.8	1:04.2	1:04.5	1:04.9	1:05.2	1:05.6	1:05.9	1:06.3
2900	1:02.0	1:02.4	1:02.7	1:03.1	1:03.4	1:03.7	1:04.1	1:04.4	1:04.8	1:05.1
2950	1:01.0	1:01.3	1:01.6	1:02.0	1:02.3	1:02.7	1:03.0	1:03.3	1:03.7	1:04.0
3000	1:00.0	1:00.3	1:00.6	1:01.0	1:01.3	1:01.6	1:02.0	1:02.3	1:02.6	1:03.0

Cruise Times Chart

25	50	75	100	150	200	250	300	350	400	450	500
:49.0	1:38.5	2:27	3:17	4:55	6:34	8:12	9:51	11:29	13:08	14:46	16:25
:49.0	1:38.0	2:27	3:16	4:54	6:32	8:10	9:48	11:26	13:04	14:42	16:20
:48.5	1:37.5	2:26	3:15	4:52	6:30	8:07	9:45	11:22	13:00	14:37	16:15
:48.5	1:37.0	2:25	3:14	4:51	6:28	8:05	9:42	11:19	12:56	14:33	16:10
:47.5	1:35.5	2:23	3:11	4:46	6:22	7:57	9:33	11:08	12:44	14:19	15:55
:47.0	1:34.0	2:21	3:08	4:42	6:16	7:50	9:24	10:58	12:32	14:06	15:40
:46.0	1:32.5	2:18	3:05	4:37	6:10	7:42	9:15	10:47	12:20	13:52	15:25
:45.5	1:31.0	2:16	3:02	4:33	6:04	7:35	9:06	10:37	12:08	13:39	15:10
:45.0	1:30.0	2:15	3:00	4:30	6:00	7:30	9:00	10:30	12:00	13:30	15:00
:44.0	1:28.5	2:12	2:57	4:25	5:54	7:22	8:51	10:19	11:48	13:16	14:45
:43.5	1:27.0	2:10	2:54	4:21	5:48	7:15	8:42	10:09	11:36	13:03	14:30
:42.5	1:25.5	2:08	2:51	4:16	5:42	7:07	8:33	9:58	11:24	12:49	14:15
:42.5	1:25.0	2:07	2:50	4:15	5:40	7:05	8:30	9:55	11:20	12:45	14:10
:41.5	1:23.5	2:05	2:47	4:10	5:34	6:57	8:21	9:44	11:08	12:31	13:55
:41.0	1:22.5	2:03	2:45	4:07	5:30	6:52	8:15	9:37	11:00	12:22	13:45
:40.5	1:21.0	2:01	2:42	4:03	5:24	6:45	8:06	9:27	10:48	12:09	13:30
:40.0	1:20.0	2:00.0	2:40	4:00	5:20	6:40	8:00	9:20	10:40	12:00	13:20
:39.0	1:18.5	1:57.5	2:37	3:55	5:14	6:32	7:51	9:09	10:28	11:46	13:05
:38.5	1:17.5	1:56.0	2:35	3:52	5:10	6:27	7:45	9:02	10:20	11:37	12:55
:38.0	1:16.0	1:54.0	2:32	3:48	5:04	6:20	7:36	8:52	10:08	11:24	12:40
:37.5	1:15.0	1:52.5	2:30	3:45	5:00	6:15	7:30	8:45	10:00	11:15	12:30
:37.0	1:14.0	1:51.0	2:28	3:42	4:56	6:10	7:24	8:38	9:52	11:06	12:20
:36.5	1:13.0	1:49.5	2:26	3:39	4:52	6:05	7:18	8:31	9:44	10:57	12:10
:36.0	1:12.0	1:48.0	2:24	3:36	4:48	6:00	7:12	8:24	9:36	10:48	12:00
:35.5	1:11.0	1:46.5	2:22	3:33	4:44	5:55	7:06	8:17	9:28	10:39	11:50
:35.0	1:10.0	1:45.0	2:20	3:30	4:40	5:50	7:00	8:10	9:20	10:30	11:40
:34.0	1:08.5	1:42.5	2:17	3:25	4:34	5:42	6:51	7:59	9:08	10:16	11:25
:33.5	1:07.5	1:41.0	2:15	3:22	4:30	5:37	6:45	7:52	9:00	10:07	11:15

11:05	9:58	8:52	7:45	6:39	5:32	4:26	3:19	2:13	1:39.5	1:06.5	:33.0
11:00	9:54	8:48	7:42	6:36	5:30	4:24	3:18	2:12	1:39.0	1:06.0	:33.0
10:50	9:45	8:40	7:35	6:30	5:25	4:20	3:15	2:10	1:37.5	1:05.0	:32.5
10:40	9:36	8:32	7:28	6:24	5:20	4:16	3:12	2:08	1:36.0	1:04.0	:32.0
10:30	9:27	8:24	7:21	6:18	5:15	4:12	3:09	2:06	1:34.5	1:03.0	:31.5
10:20	9:18	8:16	7:14	6:12	5:10	4:08	3:06	2:04	1:33.0	1:02.0	:31.0
10:10	9:09	8:08	7:07	6:06	5:05	4:04	3:03	2:02	1:31.5	1:01.0	:30.5
10:00	9:00	8:00	7:00	6:00	5:00	4:00	3:00	2:00	1:30.0	1:00.0	:30.0
9:50	8:51	7:52	6:53	5:54	4:55	3:56	2:57	1:58	1:28.5	:59.0	:29.5
9:40	8:42	7:44	6:46	5:48	4:50	3:52	2:54	1:56	1:27.0	:58.0	:29.0
9:30	8:33	7:36	6:39	5:42	4:45	3:48	2:51	1:54	1:25.5	:57.0	:28.5
9:20	8:24	7:28	6:32	5:36	4:40	3:44	2:48	1:52	1:24.0	:56.0	:28.0
9:10	8:15	7:20	6:25	5:30	4:35	3:40	2:45	1:50	1:22.5	:55.0	:27.5
9:05	8:10	7:16	6:21	5:27	4:32	3:38	2:43	1:49	1:21.5	:54.5	:27.0
9:00	8:06	7:12	6:18	5:24	4:30	3:36	2:42	1:48	1:21.0	:54.0	:27.0
8:50	7:57	7:04	6:11	5:18	4:25	3:32	2:39	1:46	1:19.5	:53.0	:26.5
8:45	7:52	7:00	6:07	5:15	4:22	3:30	2:37	1:45	1:18.5	:52.5	:26.0
8:40	7:48	6:56	6:04	5:12	4:20	3:28	2:36	1:44	1:18.0	:52.0	:26.0
8:35	7:43	6:52	6:00	5:09	4:17	3:26	2:34	1:43	1:17.0	:51.5	:25.5
8:30	7:39	6:48	5:57	5:06	4:15	3:24	2:33	1:42	1:16.5	:51.0	:25.5
8:25	7:34	6:44	5:53	5:03	4:12	3:22	2:31	1:41	1:15.5	:50.5	:25.0
8:20	7:30	6:40	5:50	5:00	4:10	3:20	2:30	1:40	1:15.0	:50.0	:25.0
8:15	7:25	6:36	5:46	4:57	4:07	3:18	2:28	1:39	1:14.0	:49.5	:24.5
8:10	7:21	6:32	5:43	4:54	4:05	3:16	2:27	1:38	1:13.5	:49.0	:24.5
8:05	7:16	6:28	5:39	4:51	4:02	3:14	2:25	1:37	1:12.5	:48.5	:24.0
8:00	7:12	6:24	5:36	4:48	4:00	3:12	2:24	1:36	1:12.0	:48.0	:24.0
7:55	7:07	6:20	5:32	4:45	3:57	3:10	2:22	1:35	1:11.0	:47.5	:23.5
7:50	7:03	6:16	5:29	4:42	3:55	3:08	2:21	1:34	1:10.5	:47.0	:23.5
7:45	6:58	6:12	5:25	4:39	3:52	3:06	2:19	1:33	1:09.5	:46.5	:23.0
7:40	6:54	6:08	5:22	4:36	3:50	3:04	2:18	1:32	1:09.0	:46.0	:23.0
7:35	6:49	6:04	5:18	4:33	3:47	3:02	2:16	1:31	1:08.0	:45.5	:22.5
7:30	6:45	6:00	5:15	4:30	3:45	3:00	2:15	1:30	1:07.5	:45.0	:22.5
7:25	6:40	5:56	5:11	4:27	3:42	2:58	2:13	1:29	1:06.5	:44.5	:22.0

(continued)

Cruise Times Chart (continued)

25	50	75	100	150	200	250	300	350	400	450	500
:22.0	:44.0	1:06.0	1:28	2:12	2:56	3:40	4:24	5:08	5:52	6:36	7:20
:21.5	:43.5	1:05.0	1:27	2:10	2:54	3:37	4:21	5:04	5:48	6:31	7:15
:21.5	:43.0	1:04.5	1:26	2:09	2:52	3:35	4:18	5:01	5:44	6:27	7:10
:21.0	:42.5	1:03.5	1:25	2:07	2:50	3:32	4:15	4:57	5:40	6:22	7:05
:21.0	:42.0	1:03.0	1:24	2:06	2:48	3:30	4:12	4:54	5:36	6:18	7:00
:20.5	:41.5	1:02.0	1:23	2:04	2:46	3:27	4:09	4:50	5:32	6:13	6:55
:20.5	:41.0	1:01.5	1:22	2:03	2:44	3:25	4:06	4:47	5:28	6:09	6:50
:20.0	:40.5	1:00.5	1:21	2:01	2:42	3:22	4:03	4:43	5:24	6:04	6:45
:20.0	:40.0	1:00.0	1:20	2:00.0	2:40	3:20	4:00	4:40	5:20	6:00	6:40
:19.5	:39.5	:59.0	1:19	1:58.5	2:38	3:17	3:57	4:36	5:16	5:55	6:35
:19.5	:39.0	:58.5	1:18	1:57.0	2:36	3:15	3:54	4:33	5:12	5:51	6:30
:19.0	:38.5	:57.5	1:17	1:55.5	2:34	3:12	3:51	4:29	5:08	5:46	6:25
:19.0	:38.0	:57.0	1:16	1:54.0	2:32	3:10	3:48	4:26	5:04	5:42	6:20
:18.5	:37.5	:56.0	1:15	1:52.5	2:30	3:07	3:45	4:22	5:00	5:37	6:15
:18.5	:37.0	:55.5	1:14	1:51.0	2:28	3:05	3:42	4:19	4:56	5:33	6:10
:18.0	:36.5	:54.5	1:13	1:49.5	2:26	3:02	3:39	4:15	4:52	5:28	6:05
:18.0	:36.0	:54.0	1:12	1:48.0	2:24	3:00	3:36	4:12	4:48	5:24	6:00
:17.5	:35.5	:53.0	1:11	1:46.5	2:22	2:57	3:33	4:08	4:44	5:19	5:55
:17.5	:35.0	:52.5	1:10	1:45.0	2:20	2:55	3:30	4:05	4:40	5:15	5:50
:17.0	:34.5	:51.5	1:09	1:43.5	2:18	2:52	3:27	4:01	4:36	5:10	5:45
:17.0	:34.0	:51.0	1:08	1:42.0	2:16	2:50	3:24	3:58	4:32	5:06	5:40
:16.5	:33.5	:50.0	1:07	1:40.5	2:14	2:47	3:21	3:54	4:28	5:01	5:35
:16.0	:32.5	:48.5	1:05	1:37.5	2:10	2:42	3:15	3:47	4:20	4:52	5:25
:16.0	:32.0	:48.0	1:04	1:36.0	2:08	2:40	3:12	3:44	4:16	4:48	5:20
:15.5	:31.5	:47.0	1:03	1:34.5	2:06	2:37	3:09	3:40	4:12	4:43	5:15
:15.5	:31.0	:46.5	1:02	1:33.0	2:04	2:35	3:06	3:37	4:08	4:39	5:10
:15.0	:30.5	:45.5	1:01	1:31.5	2:02	2:32	3:03	3:33	4:04	4:34	5:05
:15.0	:30.0	:45.0	1:00	1:30.0	2:00.0	2:30	3:00	3:30	4:00	4:30	5:00

Cruise Interval Chart

CPace (per 100)	Cruise interval											
	25	50	75	100	150	200	250	300	350	400	450	500
3:08	:55-45	1:45-30	2:35-17	3:20-07	5:00-41	6:40-16	8:20-50	9:55-24	11:35-58	13:15-32	14:55-06	16:30-40
3:06	:55-44	1:45-29	2:30-18	3:20-02	5:00-36	6:35-12	8:15-45	9:50-18	11:30-51	13:05-24	14:45-57	16:20-30
3:04	:55-44	1:40-31	2:30-15	3:20-00	4:55-35	6:30-08	8:10-40	9:45-12	11:20-44	13:00-16	14:35-48	16:10-20
3:02	:55-43	1:40-28	2:30-12	3:15-01	4:50-32	6:25-04	8:05-35	9:40-06	11:15-37	12:50-08	14:25-39	16:00-10
3:00	:50-44	1:40-26	2:25-14	3:15-55	4:50-27	6:25-00	8:00-30	9:30-00	11:05-30	12:40-00	14:15-30	15:50-00
2:58	:50-43	1:40-25	2:25-10	3:10-56	4:45-26	6:20-56	7:50-25	9:25-54	11:00-23	12:35-52	14:05-21	15:40-50
2:56	:50-42	1:35-27	2:25-08	3:10-52	4:40-23	6:15-52	7:45-20	9:20-48	10:50-16	12:25-44	13:55-12	15:30-40
2:54	:50-41	1:35-24	2:20-09	3:10-49	4:40-18	6:10-48	7:40-15	9:15-42	10:45-09	12:15-36	13:45-03	15:20-30
2:52	:50-41	1:35-23	2:20-06	3:05-50	4:35-17	6:05-44	7:35-10	9:05-36	10:35-02	12:05-28	13:40-54	15:10-20
2:50	:50-40	1:35-22	2:20-04	3:05-46	4:35-12	6:00-40	7:30-05	9:00-30	10:30-55	12:00-20	13:30-45	15:00-10
2:48	:50-40	1:35-21	2:15-05	3:00-46	4:30-11	6:00-36	7:25-00	8:55-24	10:20-48	11:50-12	13:20-36	15:00-00
2:46	:50-39	1:30-22	2:15-01	3:00-42	4:25-08	5:55-32	7:20-55	8:50-18	10:15-41	11:40-04	13:10-27	14:45-00
2:44	:50-39	1:30-20	2:15-59	2:55-42	4:25-04	5:50-28	7:15-50	8:40-12	10:10-34	11:35-56	13:00-18	14:35-50
2:42	:50-38	1:30-18	2:15-58	2:55-38	4:20-02	5:45-24	7:10-45	8:35-06	10:00-27	11:25-48	12:50-09	14:25-40
2:40	:45-39	1:30-17	2:10-58	2:55-35	4:15-59	5:40-20	7:05-40	8:30-00	9:55-20	11:15-40	12:40-00	14:15-40
2:38	:45-38	1:30-16	2:10-55	2:50-36	4:15-52	5:35-16	7:00-35	8:25-54	9:45-13	11:10-32	12:30-51	14:05-20
2:36	:45-37	1:25-17	2:10-52	2:50-32	4:10-53	5:35-12	6:55-30	8:15-48	9:40-06	11:00-24	12:20-42	13:55-10
2:34	:45-36	1:25-14	2:05-52	2:45-30	4:05-47	5:25-04	6:45-20	8:05-36	9:25-52	10:45-08	12:05-24	13:45-00
2:32	:45-36	1:25-12	2:05-49	2:45-26	4:00-44	5:20-58	6:40-15	8:00-30	9:15-45	10:35-00	11:55-15	13:25-40
2:30	:45-35	1:25-11	2:00-49	2:40-26	4:00-38	5:15-55	6:35-10	7:50-24	9:10-38	10:25-52	11:45-06	13:15-30
2:28	:45-35	1:20-12	2:00-46	2:40-22	3:55-38	5:15-51	6:30-05	7:45-18	9:00-31	10:20-44	11:35-57	13:00-20
2:26	:45-34	1:20-10	2:00-44	2:35-22	3:50-35	5:10-51	6:25-00	7:40-12	8:55-24	10:10-36	11:25-48	12:50-10
2:24	:45-34	1:20-08	1:55-45	2:35-18	3:50-29	5:05-47	6:20-55	7:40-12	8:45-17	10:00-28	11:15-39	12:40-00
2:22	:40-35	1:20-07	1:55-42	2:30-19	3:45-29	5:05-41	6:15-50	7:30-06	8:40-10	9:55-20	11:05-30	12:30-50
2:20	:40-34	1:55-42	1:55-42	2:30-19	3:45-29	5:00-39	6:15-50	7:25-00	8:40-10	9:55-20	11:05-30	12:20-40
2:18	:40-33	1:15-08	1:55-39	2:30-15	3:40-26	4:55-35	6:05-45	7:20-54	8:30-03	9:45-12	10:55-21	12:10-30

(continued)

Cruise Interval Chart (continued)

CPace (per 100)	Cruise interval 25	50	75	100	150	200	250	300	350	400	450	500
2:16	:40-32	1:15-06	1:50-40	2:30-12	3:40-20	4:50-31	6:00-40	7:15-48	8:25-56	9:35-04	10:50-12	12:00-20
2:14	:40-32	1:15-04	1:50-37	2:25-13	3:35-20	4:45-27	5:55-35	7:05-42	8:15-49	9:30-56	10:40-03	11:50-10
2:12	:40-31	1:15-03	1:50-35	2:25-09	3:35-14	4:40-23	5:50-30	7:00-36	8:10-42	9:20-48	10:30-54	11:40-00
2:10	:40-31	1:15-02	1:45-36	2:20-05	3:30-14	4:40-17	5:45-25	6:55-30	8:05-35	9:10-40	10:20-45	11:30-50
2:08	:40-30	1:10-03	1:45-33	2:20-05	3:25-11	4:35-15	5:40-20	6:50-24	7:55-28	9:05-32	10:10-36	11:15-40
2:06	:40-30	1:10-01	1:45-31	2:15-05	3:25-05	4:30-11	5:35-15	6:40-18	7:50-21	8:55-24	10:00-27	11:05-30
2:04	:40-29	1:10-00	1:45-29	2:15-01	3:20-05	4:25-07	5:30-10	6:35-12	7:40-14	8:45-16	9:50-18	10:55-20
2:02	:35-30	1:10-59	1:40-30	2:15-58	3:15-02	4:20-03	5:25-05	6:30-06	7:35-07	8:35-08	9:40-09	10:45-10
2:00	:35-29	1:10-57	1:40-27	2:10-58	3:15-55	4:15-59	5:20-58	6:25-00	7:25-00	8:30-00	9:30-00	10:35-00
1:59	:35-28	1:05-58	1:40-26	2:10-55	3:10-57	4:15-53	5:15-56	6:20-57	7:20-57	8:25-56	9:25-56	10:30-55
1:58	:35-28	1:05-57	1:40-25	2:10-53	3:10-53	4:15-51	5:15-52	6:15-54	7:20-53	8:20-52	9:25-51	10:25-50
1:57	:35-28	1:05-56	1:35-26	2:10-52	3:10-50	4:10-53	5:10-51	6:15-51	7:15-50	8:15-48	9:20-47	10:20-45
1:56	:35-28	1:05-55	1:35-24	2:05-54	3:10-49	4:10-47	5:10-47	6:10-48	7:10-46	8:10-44	9:15-42	10:15-40
1:55	:35-27	1:05-55	1:35-23	2:05-52	3:05-51	4:05-49	5:05-46	6:05-45	7:10-43	8:10-40	9:10-38	10:10-35
1:54	:35-27	1:05-54	1:35-22	2:05-49	3:05-47	4:05-43	5:05-42	6:05-42	7:05-39	8:05-36	9:05-33	10:05-30
1:53	:35-27	1:05-54	1:35-21	2:05-48	3:05-44	4:00-45	5:00-41	6:00-39	7:00-36	8:00-32	9:00-29	10:00-25
1:52	:35-27	1:05-53	1:35-21	2:05-48	3:00-46	4:00-40	5:00-37	6:00-36	6:55-32	7:55-28	8:55-24	9:55-20
1:51	:35-26	1:05-53	1:30-22	2:00-49	3:00-42	4:00-38	4:55-36	5:55-33	6:55-29	7:50-24	8:50-20	9:50-15
1:50	:35-26	1:05-52	1:30-20	2:00-47	3:00-40	3:55-39	4:55-32	5:50-30	6:50-25	7:45-20	8:45-15	9:45-10
1:49	:35-26	1:00-53	1:30-18	2:00-45	2:55-42	3:55-34	4:50-31	5:50-27	6:45-22	7:45-16	8:40-11	9:35-05
1:48	:35-26	1:00-52	1:30-18	2:00-44	2:55-38	3:50-35	4:50-27	5:45-24	6:40-18	7:40-12	8:35-06	9:30-00
1:47	:35-25	1:00-51	1:30-17	1:55-45	2:55-36	3:50-30	4:45-26	5:40-21	6:40-15	7:35-08	8:30-02	9:25-55
1:46	:35-25	1:00-50	1:30-16	1:55-43	2:50-37	3:50-28	4:45-22	5:40-18	6:35-11	7:30-04	8:25-57	9:20-50
1:45	:35-25	1:00-50	1:30-16	1:55-41	2:50-34	3:45-29	4:40-21	5:35-15	6:30-08	7:25-00	8:20-53	9:15-45
1:44	:30-25	1:00-49	1:25-17	1:55-40	2:50-31	3:45-24	4:40-17	5:35-12	6:25-04	7:20-56	8:15-48	9:10-40
1:43	:30-25	1:00-49	1:25-15	1:55-39	2:45-33	3:40-25	4:35-16	5:30-09	6:25-01	7:20-52	8:10-44	9:05-35
1:42	:30-24	1:00-48	1:25-13	1:50-40	2:45-29	3:40-20	4:35-12	5:25-06	6:20-57	7:15-48	8:05-39	9:00-30

1:41	:30-24	1:00-48	1:25-13	1:50-38	2:45-27	3:35-21	4:30-11	5:25-03	6:15-54	7:10-44	8:00-35	8:55-25
1:40	:30-24	1:00-48	1:25-12	1:50-36	2:45-26	3:35-16	4:30-08	5:20-58	6:15-50	7:05-40	8:00-30	8:50-20
1:39	:30-24	:55-48	1:25-11	1:50-35	2:40-27	3:35-14	4:25-06	5:15-56	6:10-47	7:00-36	7:55-26	8:45-15
1:38	:30-23	:55-47	1:20-12	1:50-34	2:40-23	3:30-15	4:20-04	5:15-51	6:05-43	6:55-32	7:50-21	8:40-10
1:37	:30-23	:55-46	1:20-11	1:45-35	2:40-21	3:30-10	4:20-00	5:10-50	6:00-40	6:50-28	7:45-17	8:35-05
1:36	:30-23	:55-46	1:20-09	1:45-33	2:35-22	3:25-11	4:15-59	5:05-47	6:00-36	6:50-24	7:40-12	8:30-00
1:35	:30-23	:55-45	1:20-08	1:45-31	2:35-19	3:25-06	4:15-53	5:05-42	5:55-33	6:45-20	7:35-08	8:25-55
1:34	:30-22	:55-45	1:20-07	1:45-30	2:35-17	3:20-07	4:10-54	5:00-41	5:50-29	6:40-16	7:30-03	8:20-50
1:33	:30-22	:55-44	1:20-07	1:45-29	2:30-18	3:20-02	4:10-48	5:00-36	5:45-26	6:35-12	7:25-59	8:15-45
1:32	:30-22	:55-44	1:15-08	1:40-31	2:30-15	3:20-00	4:05-49	4:55-35	5:45-22	6:30-08	7:20-54	8:10-40
1:31	:30-22	:55-44	1:15-06	1:40-28	2:30-12	3:15-01	4:05-43	4:50-32	5:40-19	6:25-04	7:15-50	8:05-35
1:30	:30-21	:55-43	1:15-05	1:40-26	2:25-14	3:15-55	4:00-44	4:50-27	5:35-15	6:25-00	7:10-45	8:00-30
1:29	:30-21	:50-44	1:15-04	1:40-25	2:25-10	3:10-56	4:00-38	4:45-26	5:30-12	6:20-56	7:05-41	7:50-25
1:28	:30-21	:50-43	1:15-03	1:35-27	2:25-08	3:10-52	3:55-39	4:40-23	5:30-08	6:15-52	7:00-36	7:45-20
1:27	:30-21	:50-42	1:15-03	1:35-24	2:20-09	3:10-49	3:55-33	4:40-18	5:25-05	6:10-48	6:55-32	7:40-15
1:26	:30-20	:50-41	1:15-02	1:35-23	2:20-06	3:05-50	3:50-34	4:35-17	5:20-01	6:05-44	6:50-27	7:35-10
1:25	:25-21	:50-41	1:10-03	1:35-22	2:20-04	3:05-46	3:50-28	4:35-12	5:15-56	6:00-40	6:45-23	7:30-05
1:24	:25-20	:50-40	1:10-01	1:35-21	2:15-05	3:00-46	3:45-29	4:30-11	5:15-51	6:00-36	6:40-18	7:25-00
1:23	:25-20	:50-40	1:10-00	1:30-22	2:15-01	3:00-42	3:45-23	4:25-08	5:10-49	5:55-32	6:35-14	7:20-55
1:22	:25-19	:50-39	1:10-59	1:30-20	2:15-59	2:55-42	3:40-24	4:25-04	5:05-46	5:50-28	6:30-09	7:15-50
1:21	:25-19	:50-39	1:10-58	1:30-18	2:15-58	2:55-38	3:40-18	4:20-02	5:05-41	5:45-24	6:30-05	7:10-45
1:20	:25-19	:50-38	1:10-57	1:30-17	2:10-58	2:55-35	3:35-19	4:20-02	5:00-39	5:40-20	6:25-00	7:05-40
1:19	:25-19	:45-39	1:05-58	1:30-16	2:10-55	2:50-36	3:30-16	4:15-59	4:55-35	5:35-16	6:20-56	7:00-35
1:18	:25-18	:45-38	1:05-56	1:25-17	2:10-52	2:50-32	3:30-11	4:15-52	4:50-32	5:35-12	6:15-51	6:55-30
1:17	:25-18	:45-37	1:05-55	1:25-15	2:05-54	2:45-32	3:25-11	4:10-53	4:50-27	5:30-08	6:10-47	6:50-25
1:16	:25-18	:45-37	1:05-54	1:25-13	2:05-51	2:45-28	3:25-06	4:10-46	4:45-25	5:25-04	6:05-42	6:45-20
1:15	:25-18	:45-36	1:05-53	1:25-12	2:05-48	2:45-26	3:20-07	4:05-47	4:40-21	5:20-58	6:00-38	6:40-15
1:14	:25-18	:45-35	1:05-53	1:25-11	2:00-49	2:40-26	3:20-01	4:00-44	4:35-18	5:15-55	5:55-33	6:35-10
1:13	:25-17	:45-35	1:00-53	1:20-12	2:00-46	2:40-22	3:15-02	4:00-38	4:35-13	5:10-51	5:50-29	6:30-05
1:12	:25-17	:45-34	1:00-52	1:20-10	2:00-44	2:35-22	3:15-55	3:55-38	4:30-11	5:05-47	5:45-24	6:25-00
1:11	:25-17	:40-35	1:00-51	1:20-08	1:55-45	2:35-18	3:10-56	3:50-35	4:25-07	5:05-41	5:40-20	6:20-55
1:10	:25-17	:40-34	1:00-50	1:20-07	1:55-42	2:30-19	3:10-51	3:45-29	4:20-04	5:00-39	5:35-15	6:15-50

About the Author

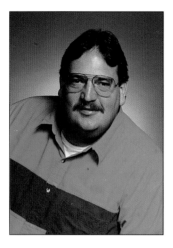

Emmett Hines is one of only nine coaches to hold the Level 5 Masters Certification—the American Swim Coaches Association's highest adult coaching certification. He has been coaching in some form since the age of 14. Since founding his company, H$_2$Ouston Swims, in 1982 he has concentrated his efforts almost exclusively on adult swimmers, from beginning swimmers all the way up to those with Olympic pedigrees. His wife Peggy runs the youth side of the swimming program. Hines is also a teaching pro at the prestigious Houstonian Club and travels the country as a senior coach and instructor trainer for Total Immersion Adult Swim Camps, the world's most widely known and respected adult swimming instruction organization.

Hines is a regularly featured writer for *Swim Magazine*, the official publication of United States Masters Swimming (USMS). He has had over 150 articles published in swimming and triathlon magazines and newsletters. He has spoken at the ASCA World Coaches Clinic and Pacific Coaches Clinic—two of the largest professional swim coaches gatherings in the world. Swimmers under his guidance have won numerous team and individual National Championship titles and have set several national and world records. Hines has served as the Assistant USMS Editor for *Swim Magazine*, editor of the Masters Aquatic Coaches Association newsletter and editor of *Gulf Masters Swimming Newsletter*. He is also an active United States Senior Olympics volunteer.